150
ECG Cases

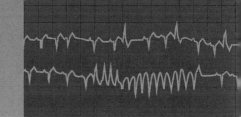

150
ECG Cases

FIFTH EDITION

JOHN HAMPTON DM MA DPhil FRCP FFPM FESC
Emeritus Professor of Cardiology, University of Nottingham, UK

DAVID ADLAM BA BM BCh DPhil FRCP FESC
Associate Professor of Acute and Interventional Cardiology and Honorary
Consultant Cardiologist, University of Leicester, UK

JOANNA HAMPTON MD MA BM BCh FRCP
Consultant Physician, Addenbrooke's Hospital, Cambridge, UK

ELSEVIER   EDINBURGH   LONDON   NEW YORK   OXFORD   PHILADELPHIA   ST LOUIS   SYDNEY   2019

ELSEVIER

First edition 1997
Second edition 2003
Third edition 2008
Fourth edition 2013
Fifth edition 2019

The right of John Hampton, David Adlam and Joanna Hampton to be identified as author(s) of this work has been asserted by them in accordance with the Copyright, Designs and Patents Act 1988.

ISBN 978-0-7020-7458-5
978-0-7020-7459-2

Printed in India
Last digit is the print number: 14   13   12   11   10   9

Content Strategist: Laurence Hunter
Content Development Specialist: Fiona Conn
Project Manager: Louisa Talbott
Design: Brian Salisbury
Illustration Manager: Karen Giacomucci
Illustrator: Helius and Chartwell Illustrators

your source for books, journals and multimedia in the health sciences
www.elsevierhealth.com

The publisher's policy is to use **paper manufactured from sustainable forests**

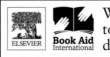

Working together to grow libraries in developing countries

www.elsevier.com • www.bookaid.org

How to use this book

Part 1 Everyday ECGs

The 75 ECGs in this section are examples of those commonly seen in clinical practice. There are several examples of the most important abnormalities, together with examples of common variations of normality. Anyone who has read *The ECG Made Easy*, 9th edition (Elsevier, 2019) should be able to interpret these ECGs correctly.

Part 2 More Challenging ECGs

The 75 ECGs in this section are more challenging and include ECG patterns seen less often, but anyone who has read *The ECG Made Practical*, 7th edition (Elsevier, 2019) should be able to interpret them.

Further Reading

These symbols indicate cross-references to useful information in *The ECG Made Easy*, 9th edition (Elsevier, 2019) and *The ECG Made Practical*, 7th edition (Elsevier, 2019).

Contents

Preface

Learning about ECG interpretation from books such as *The ECG Made Easy* or *The ECG Made Practical* (the previous editions of which were called *The ECG in Practice*) is fine so far as it goes, but it never goes far enough. As with most of medicine there is no substitute for experience, and to make the best use of the ECG there is no substitute for reviewing large numbers of them. ECGs need to be interpreted in the context of the patient from whom they were recorded. You need to learn to appreciate the variations of normality and of the patterns associated with different diseases, and to think about how the ECG can help patient management.

150 ECG Cases is the fifth edition of *150 ECG Problems*. We have changed the title to emphasize the importance of relating an ECG to the patient from whom it was recorded: these 150 records came from real patients, and at the time of recording were essential for the diagnosis and management of real patients. The aim of the book is the same as in the previous editions: it allows the inclusion of a lot more ECGs than is possible in *The ECG Made Easy* and *The ECG Made Practical*, and it is designed for the reader to improve his or her understanding of ECGs by testing recognition skills. Some 10% of the ECGs are new compared with the previous edition.

We have divided the book into two parts. The first part includes 75 ECGs that are commonly seen, and we have called this section 'Everyday ECGs' because these are the ECG patterns that crop up frequently in the Accident & Emergency department or the outpatient clinic. We have included several examples of ECGs from patients with common problems, such as myocardial infarction. Those who have read *The ECG Made Easy* should be able to recognize most of these ECGs. The second part of the book, which we have called 'More challenging ECGs' includes records seen less often, some of which could be described as 'difficult' – and in some the reader may disagree with our interpretation. But on the whole, anyone who has read *The ECG Made Practical* should get most of the ECGs in Part 2 right.

JH, DA, JH

Introduction: making the most of the ECG

Recording and reporting an ECG should never be an end in itself. The ECG is a basic and valuable tool in the investigation of cardiac problems, and it can be helpful in the case of non-cardiac problems, too, but it must always be viewed in the context of the patient from whom the record came. The ECG must never be a substitute for taking a proper medical history and carrying out a careful physical examination. Because it is simple, harmless and cheap, the ECG is usually the first investigation in a patient with possible cardiac disease, and it may be followed by the plain chest X-ray, the echocardiogram, radionuclide studies, computed tomography (CT), magnetic resonance imaging (MRI), and cardiac catheterization and angiography – but none of these are substitutes. The ECG, a recording of the electrical activity of the heart, gives information that can be obtained in no other way. However, even though it is irreplaceable, it is not infallible.

ECGs are recorded from a wide variety of patients, in an attempt to help with a wide variety of possible diagnoses. An ECG is frequently recorded in the course of 'health screening', but here it must be regarded with considerable caution. It cannot be assumed that individuals who present themselves for screening are asymptomatic – the process may be being used as a substitute for a consultation with a doctor. The ECG itself may cause difficulties of interpretation, for there are a dozen or more normal variants. Minor abnormalities, such as non-specific ST segment or T wave changes, will have diagnostic and prognostic significance if the individual has symptoms that may be cardiac in origin, but these changes can be of no importance in totally healthy people. It is rare for an ECG to demonstrate anything of importance in a totally healthy individual, although in athletes the detection of abnormalities suggesting asymptomatic hypertrophic cardiomyopathy is important.

In patients with chest pain, the ECG is important but sometimes misleading. It is essential to remember that the ECG can remain normal for some hours after the onset of a myocardial infarction. Too often patients are sent home from an A&E department because their ECG is normal, despite a reasonably convincing story of ischaemic chest pain. Under such circumstances the ECG should be repeated several times to see if changes are appearing, and patient management should depend on the plasma troponin level rather than on the ECG. Nevertheless, the ECG is important for deciding treatment in a patient with chest pain, for the management of a patient with myocardial infarction with ST segment elevation is quite different from that of a patient whose ECG shows a non-ST segment elevation infarction.

Patients with intermittent chest pain that could be angina frequently have completely normal ECGs at rest – and then the exercise test can be valuable. The exercise test is to some extent being replaced by myocardial perfusion scanning for the diagnosis of coronary disease because its predictive accuracy depends on the likelihood of the patient having angina, because there can be false negative or false positive results, and because exercise tests are sometimes unreliable in women. Remember that an exercise test is safe, but not totally safe, because arrhythmias (including ventricular fibrillation) may be induced. Nevertheless, the exercise test has the great advantage of showing a patient's exercise tolerance, and also showing what limits his capability.

The ECG also has a role in the investigation of patients with breathlessness, for it can show changes associated with heart disease (e.g. an old myocardial infarction) or with chronic chest disease. Evidence of left ventricular hypertrophy may point to hypertension, mitral regurgitation or aortic stenosis or regurgitation, and right ventricular hypertrophy may be the result of pulmonary emboli or mitral stenosis – however, all of these should have been detected during the examination of the patient. The ECG is not a good tool for grading the hypertrophy of the different heart chambers. It is particularly important to remember that the ECG cannot demonstrate heart failure: it may suggest a condition that may cause heart failure, but it is impossible to determine from an ECG whether or not a patient is in heart failure. However, in the presence of a completely normal ECG, heart failure is certainly unlikely.

There are characteristic ECG appearances in several conditions that are not primarily cardiac – for example with severe electrolyte derangement. ECG monitoring is not an acceptable way of following electrolyte changes in conditions such as diabetic ketoacidosis, but at least any abnormalities may prompt the appropriate biochemical tests. The ECG has, however, become important in the development of new drugs, for any drug that causes QT prolongation – and this is by no means uncommon – may cause sudden death due to ventricular tachycardia.

It is in the investigation and management of patients with possible arrhythmias that the ECG is of paramount importance. Patients may complain of palpitations or dizziness and syncope as a result of rhythm disturbances, and there is no way of identifying these with certainty other than with an ECG. Dizziness and syncope can be the result of rhythms that are either too fast or too slow for an effective cardiac output, or of slow rhythms associated with disorders of conduction. There may be little in the patient's history to point specifically to a cardiac problem when dizziness or collapse is the main symptom, but an appropriately abnormal ECG may immediately point to the right diagnosis. When a patient complains of palpitations there is a clearly a heart problem of some sort, and it is usually possible to come close to a diagnosis by taking a careful history – the patient with extrasystoles will describe the heart 'jumping out of the chest' or something equally unlikely, and the problem will be worse when lying down at night, and after smoking and alcohol. The patient with a true paroxysmal tachycardia will describe the sudden onset (and sometimes the sudden cessation) of the rapid heartbeat, and if the attack is associated with chest pain, dizziness or breathlessness then the presence of a paroxysmal tachycardia becomes highly likely.

Few patients will have their arrhythmia at the time they are seen, but the ECG can still give valuable clues to its nature. A patient whose ECG shows bifascicular block, or first degree atrioventricular block together with left bundle branch block, may have intermittent complete block and Stokes–Adams attacks. A patient whose ECG shows pre-excitation (the Wolff–Parkinson–White syndrome) is at risk of paroxysmal arrhythmias – though many people with these ECG patterns never have any problems at all. A patient with a prolonged QT syndrome, as a result of either a congenital defect or drug treatment, is at risk of torsade de pointes ventricular tachycardia. Under all these circumstances, ambulatory ECG recording, by one of a variety of techniques, may demonstrate the true nature of the arrhythmia that causes the symptoms – but it must be remembered that many, if not most, arrhythmias will be seen transiently in completely healthy people and only when an abnormal ECG corresponds to symptoms can one be certain that the two are related.

So the way to approach the ECG, and this book – and indeed any medical situation – is to start with the patient.

If you cannot make a reasonable diagnosis from the history, and to a lesser extent the examination, the chances of doing so as a result of investigations are not great. The role of the ECG and of more complex investigations is to help differentiate between the various possible diagnoses suggested by talking to, and examining, the patient. The clinical scenarios given with each ECG in this book are of necessity brief, but think about them, ask yourself what the diagnosis might be, and then describe and report on the ECG. That is the way to make the most of the ECG.

Part 1
Everyday ECGs

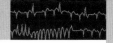

ECG 1

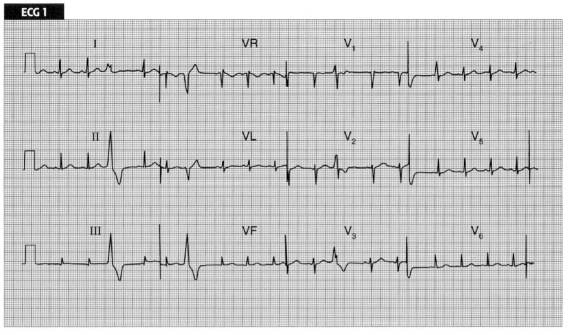

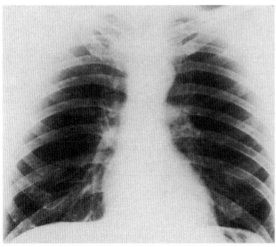

This ECG was recorded from a 20-year-old student who complained of an irregular heartbeat. Apart from an irregular pulse, her heart was clinically normal. What do the ECG and chest X-ray show and what would you do?

ANSWER 1

The ECG shows:
- Sinus rhythm, rate 100 bpm
- Ventricular extrasystoles
- Normal axis
- Normal QRS complexes and T waves

The chest X-ray is normal.

Clinical interpretation

The extrasystoles are fairly frequent, but the ECG is otherwise normal.

What to do

Ventricular extrasystoles are very common. In large groups of people, there is a correlation between the presence of extrasystoles and heart disease of many types. However, in young people who are otherwise asymptomatic and whose hearts are otherwise normal, the chances of a significant cardiac problem are very low.

Occasional extrasystoles in this context do not require investigations. With more frequent extrasystoles, an echocardiogram to confirm a structurally normal heart provides additional reassurance. Specific treatment is not usually required beyond avoidance of alcohol and caffeine.

SUMMARY

Sinus rhythm with ventricular extrasystoles.

 See *ECG Made Easy*, 9th edition, Chapter 4

ECG 2

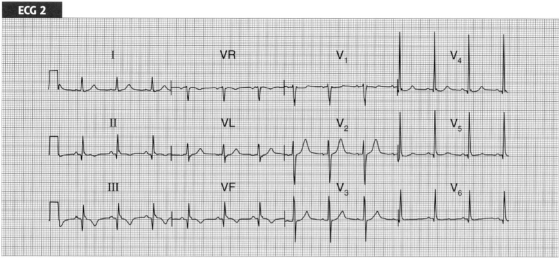

A 60-year-old man was seen as an outpatient, complaining of rather vague central chest pain on exertion. He had never had pain at rest. What does this ECG show and what would you do next?

ANSWER 2

The ECG shows:

- Sinus rhythm, rate 77 bpm
- Normal PR interval
- Normal axis
- Prominent and deep Q waves in leads II, III and VF, indicating an inferior infarction. There are also small Q waves in leads V_5–V_6, but these may be septal
- ST segments normal, with no elevation in the leads showing Q waves
- Inverted T waves in leads II, III and VF.

Clinical interpretation

The Q waves in the inferior leads, together with inverted T waves, point to an old inferior myocardial infarction.

What to do

The patient seems to have had a myocardial infarction at some point in the past, and by implication his vague chest pain may be due to angina. His coronary disease requires investigation. If he remains symptomatic on treatment consider coronary angiography. If he is asymptomatic stress MRI will allow assessment of LV function (and infarct size) as well as determining the extent of ischaemia. He will require aspirin and medical treatments to optimize risk factors, treat angina and address LV impairment if confirmed.

SUMMARY

Old inferior myocardial infarction.

 See *ECG Made Easy*, 9th edition, Chapter 5

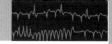

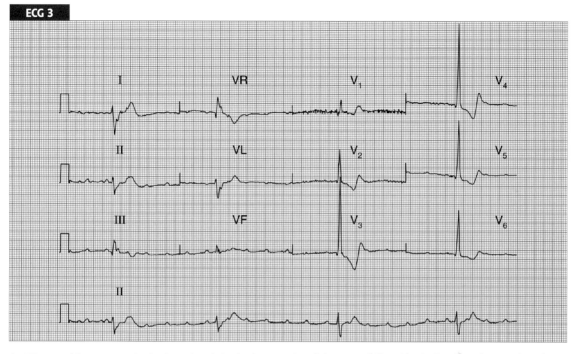

An 80-year-old woman, who had previously had a few attacks of dizziness, fell and broke her hip. She was found to have a slow pulse, and this is her ECG. The surgeons want to operate as soon as possible, but the anaesthetist is unhappy. What does the ECG show and what should be done?

ANSWER 3

The ECG shows:
- P wave rate 130 bpm
- Complete heart block
- Ventricular (QRS complex) rate 23 bpm
- The ventricular 'escape' rhythm has wide QRS complexes and abnormal T waves.

No further interpretation of the ECG is possible.

Clinical interpretation

In complete heart block there is no relationship between the P waves (here with a rate of 120 bpm) and the QRS complexes.

What to do

In the absence of a history suggesting a myocardial infarction, this woman almost certainly has chronic heart block: the fall may or may not have been due to a Stokes–Adams attack. She needs a permanent pacemaker, ideally immediately. If permanent pacing is not possible immediately, a temporary pacemaker will be needed preoperatively.

SUMMARY

Complete (third degree) heart block.

 See *ECG Made Easy*, 9th edition, Chapter 3

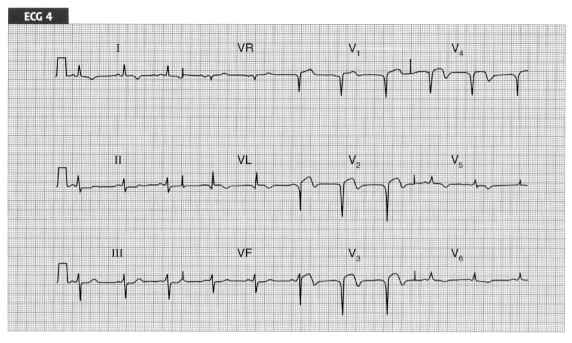

A 50-year-old man is seen in the Accident and Emergency (A&E) department with severe central chest pain which has been present for 18 h. What does this ECG show and what would you do?

ANSWER 4

The ECG shows:
- Sinus rhythm, rate 64 bpm
- Normal axis
- Q waves in leads V_2–V_4
- Raised ST segments in leads V_2–V_4
- Inverted T waves in leads I, VL, V_2–V_6.

Clinical interpretation

This is a classic acute ST segment elevation myocardial infarction (STE-ACS).

Acute coronary syndromes are subdivided into those with and without ST segment elevation (ST segment elevation ACS or STE-ACS, and non-ST segment elevation ACS or NSTE-ACS). If the troponin is raised these become ST elevation myocardial infarction (STEMI) and non-ST elevation myocardial infarction (NSTEMI). The majority of STE-ACS and some NSTE-ACS patients develop a rise in troponin, but this may be prevented by early intervention. Patients with a NSTE-ACS whose troponin remains normal are classified as having unstable angina. To be as simple as possible, and to avoid confusion, throughout this book we shall not use the terms STE-ACS and NSTE-ACS but will only describe the relevant ECGs as showing a STEMI or a NSTEMI.

What to do

More than 18 h have elapsed since the onset of pain, so this patient is outside the conventional limit for primary percutaneous coronary intervention (PCI). Nevertheless, if he is still in pain (and the pain is ischaemic rather than pericarditic in nature) and still looks unwell, PCI should be considered unless there are good reasons not to do so. If the patient is very unwell or haemodynamically compromised, consider bedside echocardiogram to exclude myocardial infarction complications (e.g. VSD, papillary muscle rupture or contained rupture). He will require treatment with dual antiplatelet therapy (with aspirin and a P2Y12 inhibitor) as soon as possible and secondary prevention therapies after revascularization.

SUMMARY

Acute anterior STEMI.

 See *ECG Made Easy*, 9th edition, Chapter 7

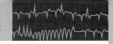
ECG 5

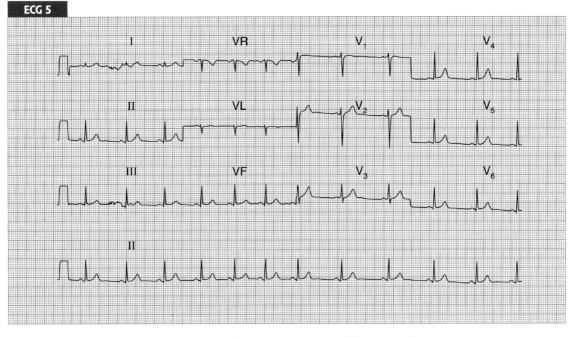

This ECG was recorded from a medical student during a practical class. What does it show?

ANSWER 5

The ECG shows:
- Sinus rhythm, rate 70 bpm
- Sinus arrhythmia
- Normal axis
- Normal QRS complexes
- Normal ST segments and T waves.

Clinical interpretation

This is a perfectly normal ECG. There is a beat-to-beat variation in the interval between QRS complexes, with the heart rate speeding up and slowing down. Comparison of the rate recorded in lead VF with that recorded in lead V$_3$ may give a false impression of a change of rhythm, but the rhythm strip (lead II) clearly shows the progressive alteration of the R–R interval. This variation in heart rate relates to respiration and is called sinus arrhythmia, which is normal in young people. Sinus arrhythmia can be distinguished from atrial extrasystoles because in sinus arrhythmia the morphology of the P waves is unchanged.

What to do

Nothing!

SUMMARY

Normal ECG with sinus arrhythmia.

 See *ECG Made Easy*, 9th edition, Chapter 2

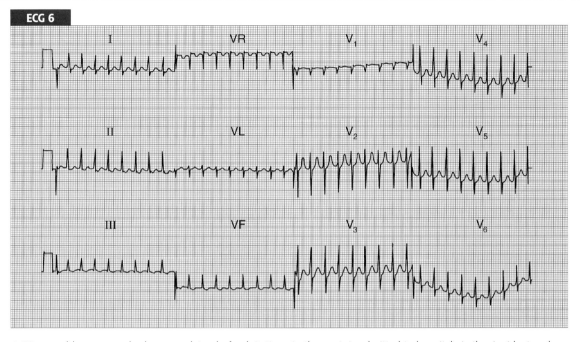

A 26-year-old woman, who has complained of palpitations in the past, is admitted to hospital via the Accident and Emergency (A&E) department with palpitations. What does the ECG show and what should you do?

ANSWER 6

The ECG shows:
- Narrow complex tachycardia, rate about 200 bpm
- No P waves visible
- Normal axis
- Regular QRS complexes
- Normal QRS complexes, ST segments and T waves.

Clinical interpretation

This is a supraventricular tachycardia, and since no P waves are visible, this is probably an atrioventricular nodal re-entry, tachycardia (AVNRT) or an atrioventricular re-entry tachycardia (AVRT).

What to do

AVNRT is the most common form of paroxysmal tachycardia in young people, and presumably explains the patient's previous episodes of palpitations. AVRT where an aberrant pathway is not evident on the resting ECG is an alternative explanation. Attacks of AVNRT or AVRT may be terminated by any of the manoeuvres that lead to vagal stimulation – Valsalva's manoeuvre, carotid sinus pressure, or immersion of the face in cold water. If these are unsuccessful, intravenous adenosine given in incremental doses should be given by bolus injection. Adenosine has a very short half-life, but can cause flushing and occasionally an asthmatic attack. If adenosine proves unsuccessful, verapamil 5–10 mg given by bolus injection will usually restore sinus rhythm. Otherwise, direct current (DC) cardioversion under sedation is indicated. If episodes are rare, prophylactic treatment may not be required but if recurrent beta-blockers or verapamil may be considered. If medical treatment is inadequate or not tolerated, specialist electrophysiological referral to consider investigations with a view to ablation treatment should be considered.

SUMMARY

Atrioventricular nodal re-entry tachycardia (AVNRT) or atrioventricular re-entry tachycardia (AVRT).

 See *ECG Made Easy*, 9th edition, Chapter 4

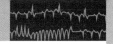

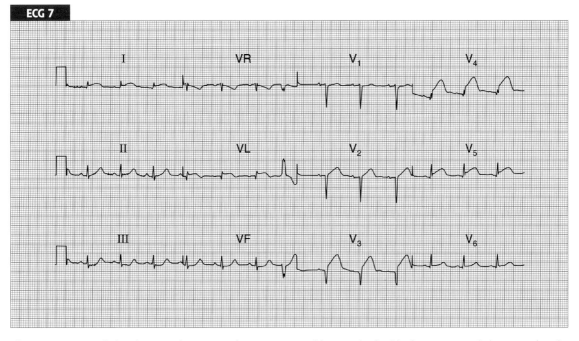

I   VR   V$_1$ V$_4$

II   VL   V$_2$ V$_5$

III   VF   V$_3$ V$_6$

This ECG was recorded in the A&E department from a 60-year-old man who had had severe central chest pain for 1 h. What does it show and what would you do?

ANSWER 7

The ECG shows:
- Sinus rhythm, rate 82 bpm
- One ventricular extrasystole
- Normal axis
- Q waves in leads V_2–V_3; small Q waves in leads VL, V_4
- Raised ST segments in leads I, VL, V_3–V_6.

Clinical interpretation

This is an acute anterolateral ST segment elevation myocardial infarction (STEMI). Although a Q wave is well developed in lead V_3, the changes are entirely consistent with the story of pain for 1 h.

What to do

The ECG shows ST segments raised by more than 2 mm in several leads, so he needs immediate primary percutaneous coronary intervention (PCI) . This treatment should not be delayed by waiting for a chest X-ray or any other investigations. This patient may need pain relief with morphine as well as dual antiplatelet therapy (usually with aspirin and a P2Y12 inhibitor) as soon as available. Ventricular extrasystoles do not need treating.

> **SUMMARY**
>
> Acute anterolateral STEMI.

 See *ECG Made Easy*, 9th edition, Chapter 7

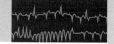

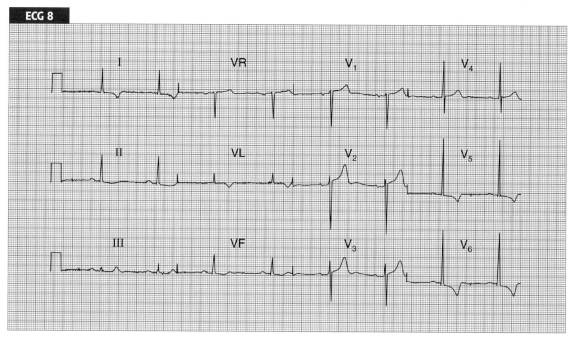

A 70-year-old retired orthopaedic surgeon telephones to say that he always gets dizzy playing golf. You find that he has a systolic heart murmur. His ECG and chest X-ray are shown. What is the diagnosis and what do you do next?

ANSWER 8

The ECG shows:
- Sinus rhythm, rate 48 bpm
- Normal axis
- QRS complex duration normal, but the R wave height in lead V_5 is 30 mm, and the S wave depth in lead V_2 is 25 mm
- Inverted T waves in leads I, VL, V_5–V_6.

The chest X-ray shows an enlarged left ventricle with 'post-stenotic' dilatation of the ascending aorta (arrowed).

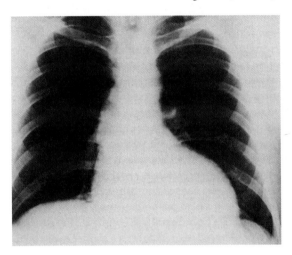 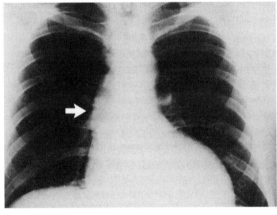

Clinical interpretation

This is the classic ECG appearance of left ventricular hypertrophy.

What to do

The combination of dizziness on exercise, a systolic murmur and evidence of left ventricular hypertrophy suggests significant aortic stenosis. The next step is an echocardiogram: in this patient it showed a gradient across the aortic valve of 140 mmHg, indicating severe stenosis. He needed an urgent aortic valve replacement.

SUMMARY

Left ventricular hypertrophy.

 See *ECG Made Easy*, 9th edition, Chapter 5

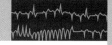

ECG 9

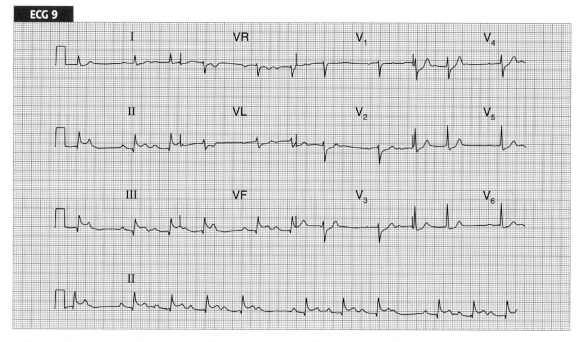

A 70-year-old man is admitted to hospital following the onset of severe central chest pain. This is his ECG. What does it show and what treatment is needed?

ANSWER 9

The ECG shows:
- Sinus rhythm, rate of sinus beats 75 bpm
- Second degree (Wenckebach) heart block (most obvious in the rhythm strip, recorded from lead II)
- Ventricular rate 70 bpm
- Normal axis
- Small Q waves in leads II, III, VF
- Raised ST segments in leads II, III, VF
- Depressed ST segments in leads V_5–V_6.

Clinical interpretation

This patient has second degree block of the Wenckebach type (progressive lengthening of the PR interval followed by a nonconducted P wave, and then a return to a short PR interval and repeat of the sequence). There is also clear evidence of a recent acute inferior ST segment elevation myocardial infarction (STEMI).

What to do

The patient should be treated in the usual way for his acute myocardial infarction, with pain relief, dual antiplatelet therapy (with aspirin and a P2Y12 inhibitor) and immediate primary percutaneous coronary intervention (PCI). Wenckebach second degree block is usually benign when it occurs with an inferior infarction, and although he must obviously be monitored until sinus rhythm with normal conduction returns, temporary pacing is not necessary.

SUMMARY

Second degree (Wenckebach) atrioventricular block with acute inferior STEMI.

 See *ECG Made Easy*, 9th edition, Chapter 3

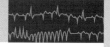

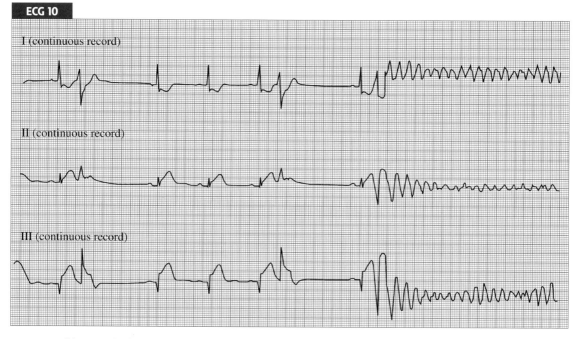

A 50-year-old man, who had come to the Accident and Emergency (A&E) department with chest pain, collapsed while his ECG was being recorded. What happened and what would you do?

ANSWER 10

The ECG shows:

- Sinus rhythm initially 55 bpm, with ventricular extrasystoles
- The third extrasystole occurs on the peak of the T wave of the preceding sinus beat
- After three or four beats of ventricular tachycardia, ventricular fibrillation develops
- In the sinus beats there is a Q wave in lead III; and there are raised ST segments in leads II and III, and ST segment depression and T wave inversion in lead I

Clinical interpretation

Although only leads I, II and III are available, it looks as if the chest pain was due to an inferior myocardial infarction. This was probably the cause of the ventricular extrasystoles, and an 'R on T' extrasystole caused ventricular tachycardia, which rapidly decayed into ventricular fibrillation. It might be argued that in lead III, and perhaps also in lead I, 'torsade de pointes' ventricular tachycardia is present, but this is not apparent in lead II.

What to do

Immediate defibrillation, but if no defibrillator is at hand then cardiopulmonary resuscitation should be performed according to advanced life support (ALS) guidelines. Following return of spontaneous circulation (ROSC) primary angioplasty is indicated.

> **SUMMARY**
>
> Probable inferior myocardial infarction; R on T ventricular extrasystole, causing ventricular fibrillation.

 See *ECG Made Easy*, 9th edition, Chapter 4

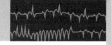

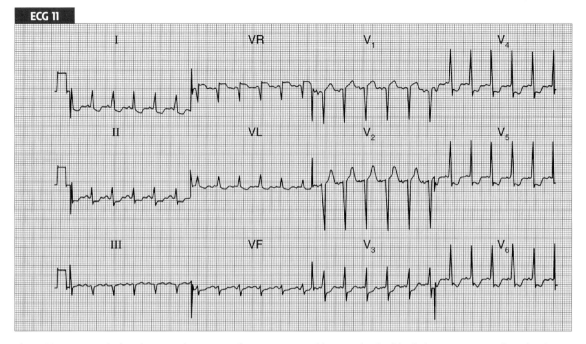

This ECG was recorded in the A&E department from a 55-year-old man who had had chest pain at rest for 6 h. There were no abnormal physical findings, and his plasma troponin level was normal. What does the trace show, and how would you manage him?

ANSWER 11

The ECG shows:
- Sinus rhythm, rate 130 bpm
- Normal axis
- Normal QRS complexes
- ST segment depression – slightly upward-sloping in lead V_3, downward-sloping in leads I, VL, V_4–V_6.

Clinical interpretation

This ECG shows anterior and lateral ischaemia without evidence of infarction. Taken with the clinical history, the diagnosis is clearly 'unstable' angina. A high sensitivity Troponin (if available) may confirm limited myocardial necrosis in keeping with a non ST elevation myocardial infarction (NSTEMI).

What to do

Given his ongoing symptoms and ischaemic ECG, this is a high risk scenario. In this context unless he settles with immediate medical treatment, urgent percutaneous coronary intervention (PCI) would probably be the treatment of choice. Immediately, dual antiplatelet therapy (with aspirin and a P2Y12 inhibitor) are indicated and sublingual or intravenous nitrates may help. A beta-blocker (if adequate blood pressure and no contra-indication) may also be considered to bring his heart rate down. Ultimately secondary prevention therapies will also be required.

> **SUMMARY**
>
> Anterolateral ischaemia.

 See *ECG Made Easy*, 9th edition, Chapter 7

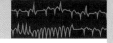
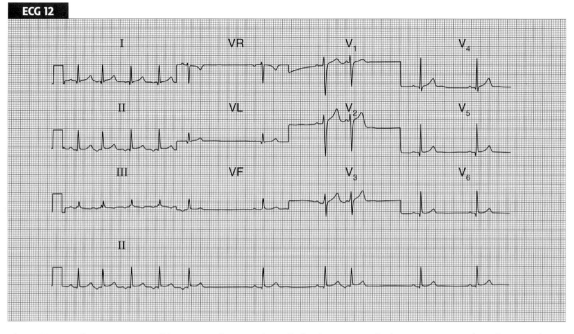

This ECG came from a 40-year-old woman who complained of palpitations, which were present when the recording was made. What abnormality does it show?

ANSWER 12

The ECG shows:
- Lead II rhythm strip of the ECG
- The first beat has a normal P wave and is normal (i.e. a sinus beat)
- The next four beats, at about 100 bpm, have abnormal (inverted) P waves, and this is an atrial tachycardia
- After a pause, the next two beats have normal P waves and are in sinus rhythm at about 60/min
- After two sinus beats, there is an extrasystole with an inverted P wave; this is an atrial extrasystole
- Normal axis
- The QRS complexes, ST segments and T waves are normal.

Clinical interpretation

Since the patient had her symptoms at the time of the recording, we can be confident that the ECG findings explain them. Atrial extrasystoles are not a manifestation of cardiac disease, but the atrial tachycardia may be and will need treating on symptomatic grounds.

What to do

Ensure that there is no other evidence of heart disease. She should stop smoking and avoid alcohol, coffee and tea. A beta-blocker will probably prevent the tachycardia.

> **SUMMARY**
>
> Sinus rhythm with atrial tachycardia and one atrial extrasystole.

 See *ECG Made Easy*, 9th edition, Chapter 4

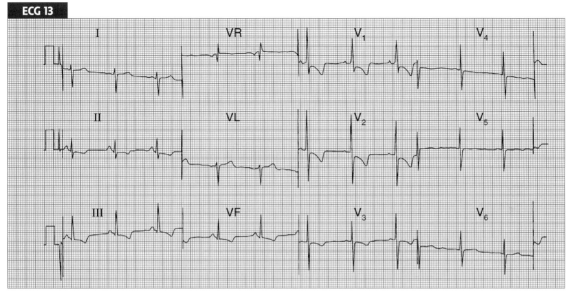

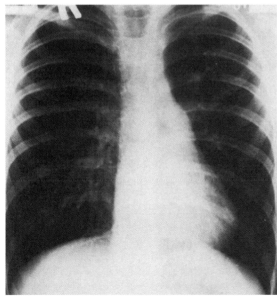

A 40-year-old woman is referred to the outpatient department because of increasing breathlessness. What do this ECG and chest X-ray show, what physical signs might you expect, and what might be the underlying problem? What might you do?

ANSWER 13

The ECG shows:

- Sinus rhythm, rate 65 bpm
- Peaked P waves, best seen in lead II
- Right axis deviation
- Dominant R waves in lead V_1
- Deep S waves in lead V_6
- Inverted T waves in leads II, III, VF, V_1–V_3.

The chest X-ray shows a slightly enlarged heart with a high cardiac apex and a prominent main pulmonary artery, suggesting right ventricular hypertrophy.

Clinical interpretation

This combination of right axis deviation, dominant R waves in lead V_1 and inverted T waves spreading from the right side of the heart is classic of severe right ventricular hypertrophy. Right ventricular hypertrophy can result from congenital heart disease, or from pulmonary hypertension, which may be idiopathic or secondary to mitral valve disease, lung disease or pulmonary embolism. The physical signs of right ventricular hypertrophy are a left parasternal heave and a displaced but diffuse apex beat. There may be a loud pulmonary second sound. The jugular venous pressure may be elevated, and a 'flicking A' wave in the jugular venous pulse is characteristic of pulmonary hypertension.

What to do

This woman requires urgent investigation to assess the underlying cause of her pulmonary hypertension. The first step will be to confirm the diagnosis by echocardiography. The two main causes of pulmonary hypertension of this degree in a 40-year-old woman are recurrent pulmonary emboli, and idiopathic (primary) pulmonary hypertension. Clinically, it is difficult to differentiate between the two, but a lung scan and computed tomography (CT) pulmonary angiography will help. In either case, anticoagulants are indicated. In fact, this patient had primary pulmonary hypertension, and treatment with high dose calcium channel blockers, prostanoids, endothelin receptor antagonists (bosentan) and phosphodiesterase inhibitors was tried, without success. Eventually she needed heart and lung transplantation.

SUMMARY

Severe right ventricular hypertrophy.

 See *ECG Made Easy*, 9th edition, Chapter 5

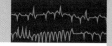

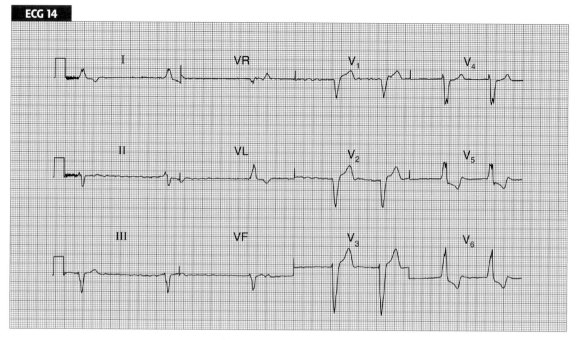

This ECG was recorded from an 80-year-old man who complained of breathlessness and ankle swelling which had become slowly worse over the preceding few months. He had had no chest pain and was on no treatment. He had a slow pulse and signs of heart failure. What does the ECG show and how would you manage him?

ANSWER 14

The ECG shows:
- Atrial fibrillation with a ventricular rate of about 40 bpm
- Left axis deviation
- Left bundle branch block (LBBB).

Clinical interpretation

When an ECG shows LBBB, no further interpretation is usually possible. Here there is atrial fibrillation, and the ventricular response is very slow, suggesting that there is conduction delay in the His bundle as well as in the left bundle branch. This could also be exacerbated by his medications (if he is taking beta-blockers, diltiazem, verapamil or digoxin).

What to do

It is always important to establish the cause of heart failure. In this patient the slow ventricular rate may be at least part of the problem. The most important causes of LBBB are ischaemia, aortic stenosis and cardiomyopathy. In this patient, an echocardiogram will show whether he has significant valve disease and how impaired his left ventricular function is. In the absence of pain, coronary angiography is probably not indicated. The heart failure needs to be treated but beta-blockers must be avoided as these may slow the ventricular response still further. If no drug-related cause for his bradycardia is identified, he almost certainly needs a permanent pacemaker. Anticoagulation should also be considered given his atrial fibrillation.

> **SUMMARY**
>
> Atrial fibrillation and LBBB.

 See *ECG Made Easy*, 9th edition, Chapter 3

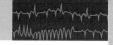

ECG 15

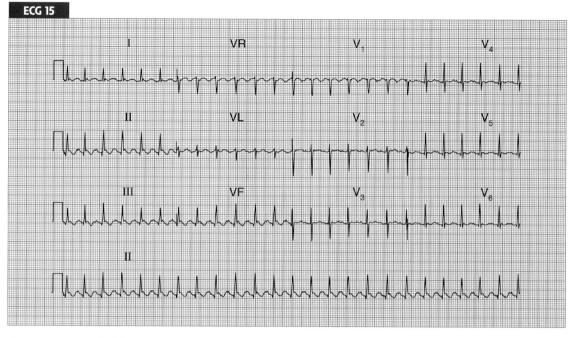

This ECG was recorded from a 40-year-old man who was admitted to hospital as an emergency, with the sudden onset of the symptoms and signs of severe left ventricular failure. What does it show and what would you do?

ANSWER 15

The ECG shows:
- Atrial flutter with 2:1 block (best seen in leads II, III, VF)
- Normal axis
- Normal QRS complexes
- The T waves are difficult to identify because of the flutter waves.

Clinical interpretation

It is a bit unusual for the onset of atrial flutter in a young and otherwise fit male to cause severe left ventricular failure. Sometimes an asymptomatic tachyarrhythmia can lead over time to impaired left ventricular function (a tachycardiomyopathy). Alternatively there may be another cause of left ventricular impairment (such as a cardiomyopathy) which has only become manifest by the onset of arrhythmia. There is nothing on the ECG to suggest a cause for the arrhythmia.

What to do

Initial treatment depends on the severity of symptoms. Milder cases may be managed initially with rate control and anticoagulation. However, when an arrhythmia causes severe heart failure immediate treatment may be necessary. In a severely compromised patient treatment under sedation with direct current (DC) cardioversion should be considered. Ideally this should be guided by transoesophageal ECHO unless the timing of onset of the arrhythmia is clear from the history and is <48 hours. This is to exclude left atrial appendage thrombus (which, if present, can be dislodged during cardioversion leading to stroke). In the long term, this patient will require further investigations and ablation therapy may be considered to prevent further episodes of atrial flutter.

> **SUMMARY**
>
> Atrial flutter with 2:1 block.

 See *ECG Made Easy*, 9th edition, Chapter 4

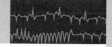

ECG 16

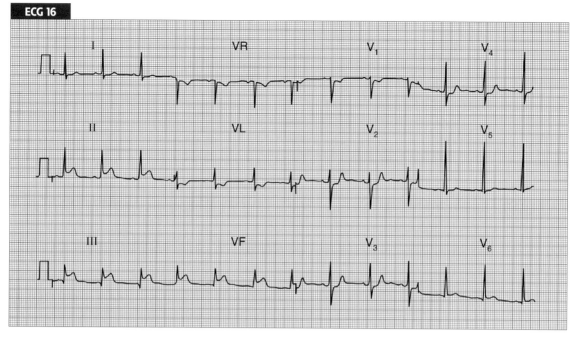

A 50-year-old man is admitted to hospital as an emergency, having had chest pain characteristic of a myocardial infarction for 4 h. Apart from the features associated with pain, there are no abnormal physical findings. What does this ECG show and what would you do?

ANSWER 16

The ECG shows:

- Sinus rhythm, rate 72 bpm
- Normal axis
- Small Q waves in lead III
- Elevated ST segments in leads II, III, VF, with upright T waves
- Suggestion of ST segment depression in leads V_2–V_3
- T wave inversion in lead VL.

Clinical interpretation

A classic ECG of an acute inferior myocardial infarction, with lead VL indicating ischaemia. The rate of development of Q waves is very variable: compare this record with ECG 32, which came from a patient with a similar duration of symptoms.

What to do

The patient should be given analgesia, dual antiplatelet therapy (with aspirin and a P2Y12 inhibitor) and referred for urgent primary percutaneous coronary intervention (PCI). Secondary prevention therapy will need to be initiated after revascularization.

SUMMARY

Acute inferior STEMI.

 See *ECG Made Easy*, 9th edition, Chapter 5

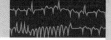

ECG 17

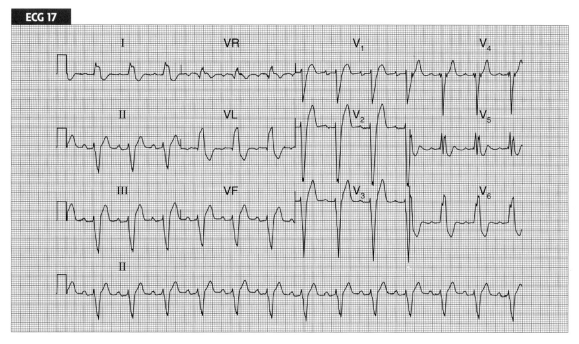

A 75-year-old woman complained of central chest discomfort on climbing hills, together with dizziness; on one occasion she had 'fainted' while climbing stairs. What abnormality does this ECG show and what physical signs would you look for?

ANSWER 17

The ECG shows:
- Sinus rhythm, rate 79 bpm
- Left axis deviation
- Broad QRS complexes (192 ms)
- 'M' pattern in lead V_6
- Inverted T waves in leads I, VL, V_6.

Clinical interpretation

This is the characteristic pattern of left bundle branch block (LBBB). The ECG cannot be interpreted further.

What to do

A patient who has chest pain that could be angina, and who has dizziness and syncope on exertion, could have severe aortic stenosis – this was the case with this woman. Clinically she had a slow rising pulse, a blood pressure of 100/80, and a slightly enlarged heart. There was a loud ejection systolic murmur, best heard at the upper right sternal edge and radiating to both carotids. The diagnosis was confirmed by an echocardiogram, which showed a gradient across the aortic valve of about 100 mmHg. A cardiac catheter was conducted to exclude coronary disease before proceeding to an aortic valve replacement.

> **SUMMARY**
>
> Sinus rhythm with LBBB.

 See *ECG Made Easy*, 9th edition, Chapter 3

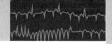

ECG 18

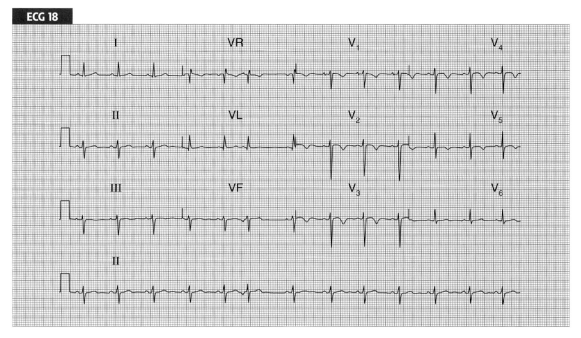

This ECG was recorded from a 48-year-old man who had had severe central chest pain for 1 h. What does it show and what would you do?

ANSWER 18

The ECG shows:
- Sinus rhythm, rate 75 bpm
- Left axis deviation (left anterior hemiblock)
- Normal QRS complexes, with a small Q wave (probably septal) in lead VL
- Inverted T waves in leads V_1–V_5.

Clinical interpretation

This is a classic acute anterior non-ST segment elevation myocardial infarction (NSTEMI).

What to do

This ECG does not meet the conventional criteria for immediate primary percutaneous coronary intervention (PCI), which are raised ST segments or new left bundle branch block. However, if symptoms persist despite initial treatment or ECG changes evolve, urgent PCI may still be required. The treatment is pain relief, dual antiplatelet therapy (aspirin and a P2Y12 inhibitor), heparin, a beta-blocker and a statin – with PCI as soon as possible. The immediate outlook is good but the patient should be monitored closely and the ECG repeated after 1 h to see if ST segment elevation is appearing.

SUMMARY

Acute anterior NSTEMI.

 See *ECG Made Easy*, 9th edition, Chapter 7

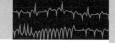
ECG 19

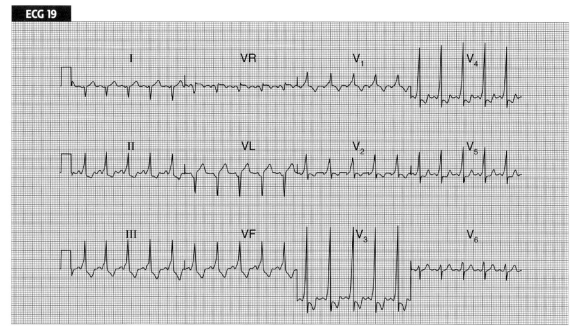

A 20-year-old student complains of palpitations. Attacks occur about once per year. They start suddenly, his heart feels very fast and regular, and he quickly feels breathless and faint. The attacks stop suddenly after a few minutes. There are no abnormalities on examination, and this is his ECG. What would you do?

ANSWER 19

The ECG shows:
- Sinus rhythm, rate 56 bpm
- Short PR interval, most obvious in the chest leads
- Normal axis
- Wide QRS complexes (136 ms)
- Slurred upstroke of the QRS complex (delta wave)
- Dominant R wave in lead V_1.

Clinical interpretation

This ECG is classic of Wolff–Parkinson–White (WPW) syndrome. The resemblance to the ECG of right ventricular hypertrophy is because this is WPW type A, with a left-sided accessory pathway.

What to do

The patient gives a clear story of a paroxysmal tachycardia, and during attacks he feels dizzy, so the circulation is clearly compromised. The attacks are infrequent, so there is little point in recording an ambulatory ECG. The patient needs immediate referral to an electrophysiologist for consideration of ablation of the aberrant conducting pathway.

> ### SUMMARY
>
> The WPW syndrome type A.

 See *ECG Made Easy*, 9th edition, Chapter 8

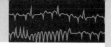

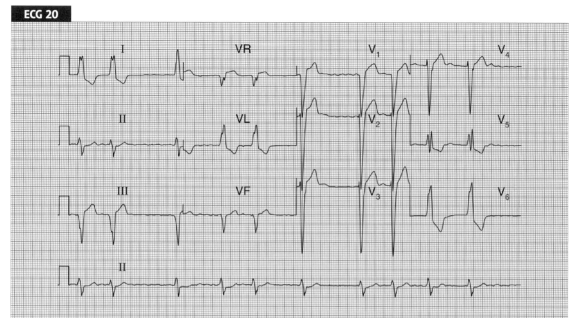

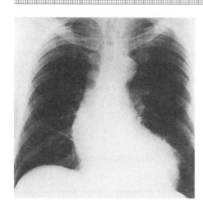

This ECG and chest X-ray are from a 70-year-old man who had had angina for some time and was being treated with a beta-blocker. He came to the A&E department complaining of pain similar to his angina, but much more severe and persistent for 4 h. He had a heart murmur. What do the ECG and chest X-ray show and what treatment would be appropriate?

ANSWER 20

The ECG shows:

- Atrial fibrillation; ventricular rate 62 bpm
- Left axis deviation (left anterior hemiblock)
- Broad QRS complexes (160 ms)
- 'M' pattern of QRS complexes in leads V_5–V_6
- Inverted T waves in leads I, VL, V_5–V_6.

The chest X-ray shows an enlarged left ventricle and a dilated ascending aorta.

Clinical interpretation

This ECG shows atrial fibrillation and left bundle branch block (LBBB). No further interpretation is possible.

What to do

The differential diagnosis in this patient is quite broad. The chest pain is perhaps most likely to be due to myocardial ischaemia or infarction. If LBBB is new, primary percutaneous coronary intervention is indicated. The dilated ascending aorta could suggest either aortic valve disease or aortic dissection. A careful history and early echocardiography are essential. However, if the chest pain is typical of his usual angina and assessments do not suggest either aortic valve disease or dissection, coronary assessment by angiography is a reasonable next step. Medical therapy will depend on the diagnosis but consideration should be given to long-term anticoagulants because of the atrial fibrillation.

> **SUMMARY**
>
> Atrial fibrillation and LBBB.

 See *ECG Made Easy*, 9th edition, Chapter 4

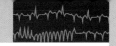

ECG 21

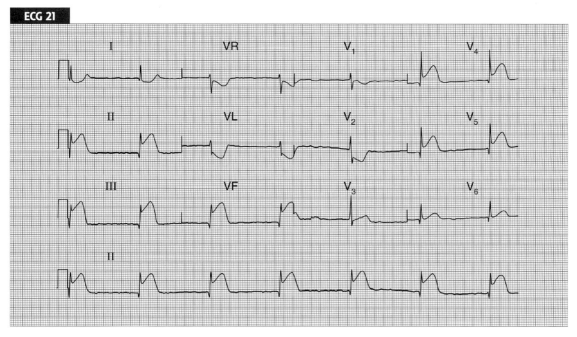

A 50-year-old man is admitted to hospital as an emergency, having had chest pain for 4 h. The pain is characteristic of a myocardial infarction. Apart from signs due to pain, the examination is normal. What does this ECG show and what would you do?

ANSWER 21

The ECG shows:
- Sinus rhythm, rate 38 bpm
- Normal axis
- Small Q waves in leads II, III, VF, V_4–V_6
- Normal QRS complexes in the chest leads
- Raised ST segments in leads II, III, VF and to a lesser extent in V_4 and V_5
- Downward-sloping ST segments in leads VL and V_2.

Clinical interpretation

This is an acute ST segment elevation inferior myocardial infarction (STEMI). The rapidity of Q wave development is extremely variable, but the trace is certainly consistent with a 4 h history. The depressed and downward-sloping ST segment in lead V_2 suggests involvement of the posterior wall of the left ventricle.

What to do

In the absence of contraindications, the patient should be given analgesia as required and dual antiplatelet therapy (aspirin and a P2Y12 inhibitor) immediately, and then proceed to primary percutaneous coronary intervention (PCI) as soon as possible.

SUMMARY

Acute inferior STEMI.

 See *ECG Made Easy*, 9th edition, Chapter 7

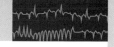

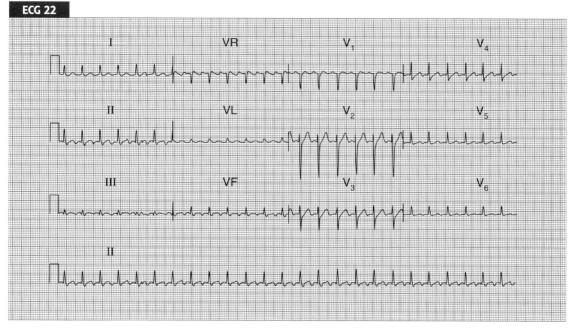

This ECG was recorded from a 40-year-old man who complained of breathlessness on climbing stairs. He was not aware of a fast heart rate and had had no chest pain. Apart from a rapid rate there were no cardiovascular abnormalities, but he looked a little jaundiced and had an enlarged spleen. What would you do?

ANSWER 22

The ECG shows:
- Atrial flutter
- Ventricular rate 148 bpm
- Normal axis
- Normal QRS complexes, ST segments and T waves.

Clinical interpretation

Atrial flutter with 2 : 1 block.

What to do

Provided the patient is not in heart failure, it is always a good idea to identify the cause of an arrhythmia before treating it. The combination of an atrial arrhythmia, jaundice and splenomegaly may suggest alcoholism, although other causes are possible. The patient needs consideration for anticoagulants, but his INR (international normalized ratio) may already be high and should be checked first. An echocardiogram is needed to assess left ventricular function. Rate control with a beta-blocker, if blood pressure allows, is a reasonable initial strategy. Long term management will depend on the cause and response to medical therapies but may include either a conservative approach with long term medication, cardioversion or ablation therapy.

> **SUMMARY**
>
> Atrial flutter with 2 : 1 conduction.

 See *ECG Made Easy*, 9th edition, Chapter 4

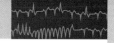

ECG 23

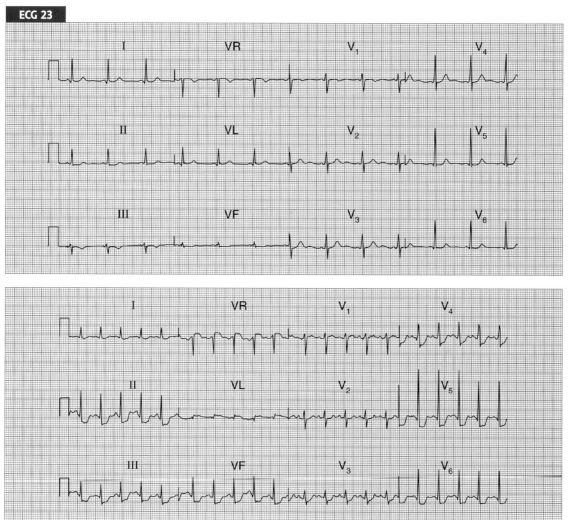

A 60-year-old man was referred to the outpatient department because of exercise-induced chest pain. The upper ECG is his record at rest, and the lower one was taken during stage 1 of the Bruce exercise protocol (1.7 mph and 10% grade on the treadmill). What do these ECGs show and what would you do?

ANSWER 23

Upper ECG

The ECG shows:

- Sinus rhythm, rate 75 bpm
- Normal axis
- Normal QRS complexes
- Slight ST segment depression in leads II, VF, V_6
- T wave inversion in lead III.

Clinical interpretation

The ST segment changes in leads II, VF and V_6 are nonspecific, and the T wave inversion in lead III could well be a normal variant. Nevertheless, with the story of exercise-induced chest pain a diagnosis of angina seems likely, and initiation of therapy and investigation to allow risk stratification are the appropriate next steps.

Lower ECG

The ECG shows:

- Sinus rhythm at 140 bpm
- Normal axis
- Normal QRS complexes
- ST segment depression in most leads, the maximum being 4 mm in lead V_5.

Clinical interpretation

Exercise ECG is used much less frequently as the primary investigation of stable patients due to the relatively high false positive and false negative rates with guidelines favouring imaging strategies. In this historical case, the resting ECG shows only nonspecific changes, but the ECG on exercise shows the classic changes of ischaemia – appearing during the first stage of the Bruce protocol. Even this light exercise level markedly increased the heart rate. Both the inferior and the anterior chest leads show definite ischaemia, so widespread coronary disease is likely, possibly including the main stem of the left coronary artery.

What to do

This patient can be treated immediately with short-acting nitrates. Presuming that the ECG changes settle, he will require admission for urgent coronary angiography with a view to percutaneous coronary intervention (PCI) or coronary artery bypass graft surgery.

SUMMARY

Nonspecific ECG changes at rest; strongly positive exercise test.

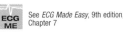

See *ECG Made Easy*, 9th edition, Chapter 7

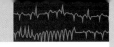

ECG 24

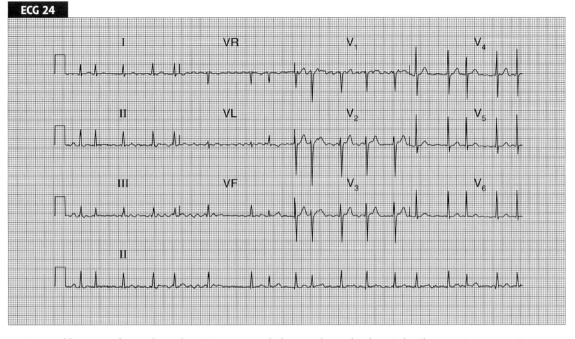

A 70-year-old woman, from whom this ECG was recorded, was admitted to hospital with increasing congestive cardiac failure. What does the ECG show and what would you do?

ANSWER 24

The ECG shows:
- Atrial fibrillation, rate about 110 bpm
- Normal axis
- Normal QRS complexes
- Normal ST segments.

Clinical interpretation

The rhythm could be interpreted as atrial flutter, particularly in lead VL. However, the flutter-like activity is variable, and the QRS complexes are completely irregular, so this is atrial fibrillation. The ST segments are normal and the ventricular rate is not controlled.

What to do

The ventricular rate in this case is rapid, and the uncontrolled rate may be contributing to the patient's heart failure. Her thyroid function tests should be checked, and she needs an echocardiogram to assess heart size and left ventricular function. The heart rate needs to be controlled and the cautious introduction of a beta-blocker should be considered. Her heart failure must be treated with a diuretic and probably an angiotensin-converting enzyme inhibitor. Anticoagulation should be considered whatever her echocardiogram shows.

SUMMARY

Atrial fibrillation with an uncontrolled ventricular rate.

 See *ECG Made Easy*, 9th edition, Chapter 4

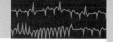

ECG 25

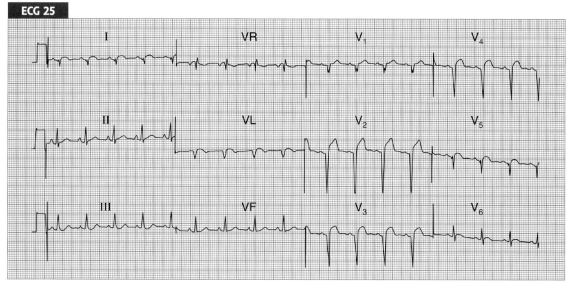

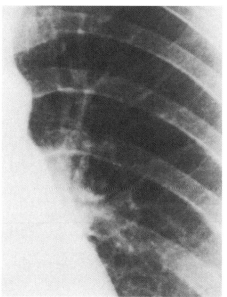

A 70-year-old man was seen as an outpatient with symptoms and signs of heart failure. His problem had begun quite suddenly a few weeks previously, when he had had a few hours of dull central chest discomfort. What do his ECG and the enlarged part of his chest X-ray show and what would you do?

ANSWER 25

The ECG shows:
- Sinus rhythm, rate 100 bpm
- Normal axis
- Q waves in leads I, VL, V_2–V_5
- Raised ST segments in leads I, VL, V_2–V_6.

The chest X-ray shows diversion of blood flow to the upper zones of the lungs, which is an early radiological sign of heart failure.

Clinical interpretation

The raised ST segments suggest an acute infarction, but the deep Q waves suggest that the infarction occurred at least several hours previously. From the patient's story it seems clear that he had an infarction several weeks before he was seen, and there was nothing in the history to suggest a more recent episode. These ECG changes are therefore probably all old; the anterior changes might indicate a left ventricular aneurysm.

What to do

An ECG should always be interpreted in the light of the patient's clinical state. Since the ECG and clinical presentation is compatible with an old infarction it should be assumed that this diagnosis is correct, and the patient should be treated for heart failure in the usual way with diuretics, angiotensin-converting enzyme inhibitors and beta-blockers. Since the heart failure is clearly due to ischaemia, he also needs aspirin and a statin. Once medically stabilized, consideration can be given to cardiac stress MRI to assess LV function (and the extent of infarction) and the extent of any residual ischaemia.

> **SUMMARY**
>
> Anterolateral myocardial infarction of uncertain age.

 See *ECG Made Easy*, 9th edition, Chapter 7

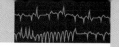

ECG 26

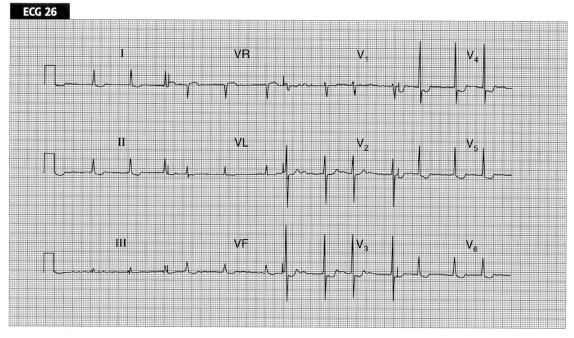

An 80-year-old woman, who has apparently been treated for heart failure for years, complains of nausea and vomiting. No previous records are available. Does her ECG help her management?

ANSWER 26

The ECG shows:
- Atrial fibrillation, ventricular rate 80 bpm
- Normal axis
- Normal QRS complexes
- Downward-sloping ST segment depression, especially in leads V_4–V_6
- T waves probably upright
- Prominent U waves in leads V_2–V_3.

Clinical interpretation

The ECG shows atrial fibrillation with a controlled ventricular rate. There is nothing on the ECG to suggest a cause for the arrhythmia or the patient's heart failure. The 'reversed tick' ST segment depression suggests that she is being treated with digoxin. The ECG does not suggest digoxin toxicity, but nevertheless this is a potential cause of her nausea. The U waves may be normal, but raise the possibility of hypokalaemia.

What to do

Digoxin is not generally used as first-line rate controlling treatment but it may be that alternatives have already been tried unsuccessfully. Measures of her plasma potassium and digoxin levels should certainly be checked and her treatment adjusted accordingly.

SUMMARY

Atrial fibrillation and digoxin effect.

 See *ECG Made Easy*, 9th edition, Chapter 5

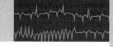

ECG 27

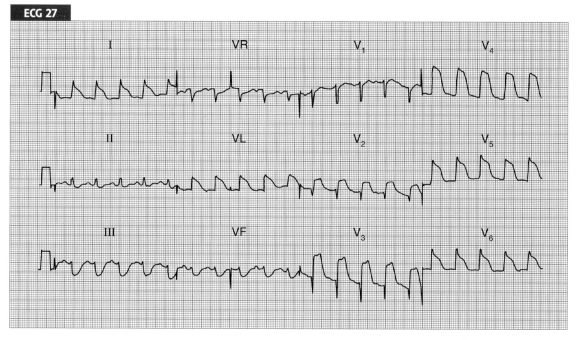

This ECG was recorded from a 65-year-old woman admitted to hospital as an emergency because of severe chest pain for 1 h. What does the ECG show? What other investigations would you order?

ANSWER 27

The ECG shows:

- Sinus rhythm, rate 111 bpm
- Normal axis
- Probably normal QRS complexes
- Gross elevation of ST segments in anterior and lateral leads
- Depressed ST segments in the inferior leads (III, VF).

Clinical interpretation

Acute ST segment elevation anterolateral myocardial infarction (STEMI). In the lateral leads I, VL and V_4–V_6, it is difficult to see where the QRS complexes end and the ST segments begin, but in lead II it is clear that the QRS complex is of normal width.

What to do

Emergency treatment for a myocardial infarction – pain relief, dual antiplatelet therapy (aspirin and P2Y12 inhibitor) and primary percutaneous coronary intervention (PCI) – should be commenced immediately. Following revascularization, initiation of secondary prevention therapies will be required.

SUMMARY

Acute anterolateral STEMI.

 See *ECG Made Easy*, 9th edition, Chapter 7

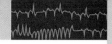

ECG 28

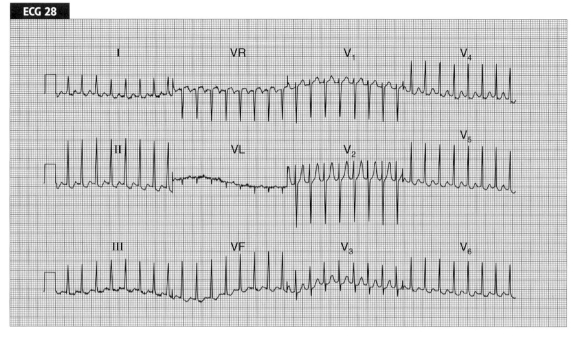

A 45-year-old woman had complained of occasional attacks of palpitations for 20 years, and eventually this ECG was recorded during an attack. What are the palpitations due to, and what would you do?

ANSWER 28

The ECG shows:
- Narrow complex tachycardia at 188 bpm
- No P waves visible
- Normal axis
- QRS complexes normal
- Some ST segment depression.

Clinical interpretation

This ECG shows supraventricular tachycardia. This rhythm is usually due to a re-entry pathway within, or near to, the atrioventricular node, so the rhythm is properly called AV nodal re-entry tachycardia (AVNRT). Alternatively an AVRT where an aberrant pathway is not evident on the resting ECG may present similarly. The ST segment depression could indicate ischaemia, but the ST segments are not horizontally depressed, nor is the depression greater than 2 mm, so it is probably of no significance.

What to do

Valsalva's manoeuvre or carotid sinus massage may be tried and will sometimes terminate the attack. If this fails, it will almost certainly respond to intravenous adenosine. Once sinus rhythm has been restored, prophylactic medication may not be needed if attacks are infrequent. Patients with recurrent problematic episodes despite medical therapy may require specialist electrophysiological assessment to consider ablation therapy.

> **SUMMARY**
>
> AV nodal re-entry (junctional) tachycardia (AVNRT).

 See *ECG Made Easy*, 9th edition, Chapter 8

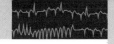

ECG 29

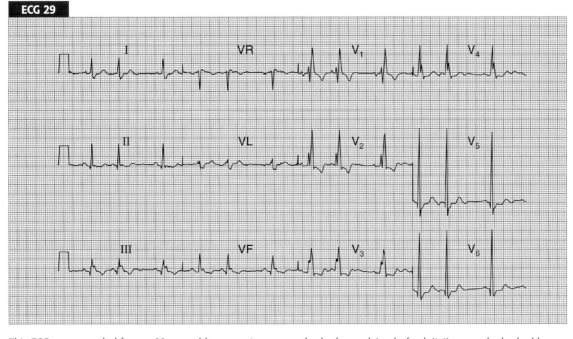

This ECG was recorded from a 23-year-old pregnant woman who had complained of palpitations, and who had been found to have a heart murmur. What does it show and what might be the problem?

ANSWER 29

The ECG shows:
- Sinus rhythm, underlying rate 61 bpm
- Supraventricular (atrial) extrasystoles
- Normal PR interval
- Normal axis
- Wide QRS complex (160 ms)
- RSR^1 pattern in lead V$_1$
- Broad slurred S wave in lead V$_6$
- Inverted T waves in leads V$_1$–V$_3$.

Clinical interpretation

The broad QRS complex with an RSR^1 pattern in lead V$_1$ and a slurred S wave in lead V$_6$, together with the inverted T waves in leads V$_1$–V$_3$, indicate right bundle branch block (RBBB). The extrasystoles are supraventricular because they have the same (abnormal) QRS pattern as the sinus beats; they are atrial in origin because each is preceded by a P wave of slightly different shape from the sinus beats.

What to do

The palpitations of which the patient complains may well be due to the extrasystoles: it is important to ensure that they correspond to her symptoms. RBBB in a young person may indicate an atrial septal defect, and she should have an echocardiogram. The heart murmur could be due to a septal defect, but could well be a 'flow murmur' due to the increased cardiac output associated with pregnancy.

SUMMARY

RBBB and atrial extrasystoles.

 See *ECG Made Easy*, 9th edition, Chapter 3

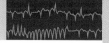

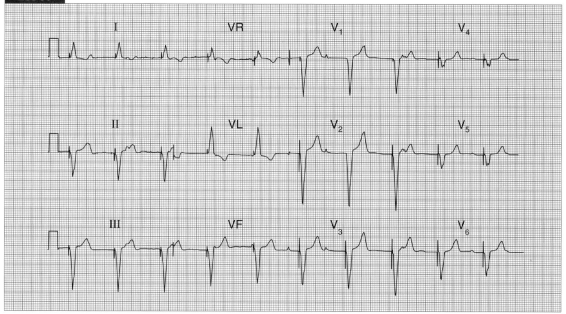

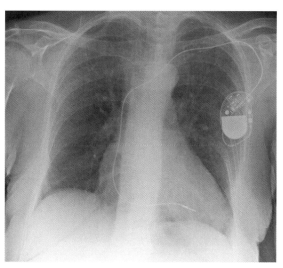

The senior house officer in the A&E department is puzzled by this ECG, which was recorded from an 80-year-old admitted unconscious with a stroke. What has the house officer missed? Perhaps he did not make a proper examination and did not look at the chest X-ray?

ANSWER 30

The ECG shows:
- Regular rhythm at 60 bpm
- Occasional P waves, not related to QRS complexes (e.g. in lead I)
- Left axis deviation
- QRS complexes preceded by a sharp 'spike'
- Broad QRS complexes (160 ms)
- Deep S wave in lead V_6
- Inverted T waves in leads I, VL.

The chest X-ray shows a permanent pacemaker, with a single lead in the right ventricle.

Clinical interpretation

The sharp spikes preceding each QRS complex are due to the pacemaker. The P waves that can occasionally be seen indicate that the underlying rhythm is complete heart block – presumably the reason why the pacemaker was inserted.

What to do

The house officer has missed the pacemaker, which is usually buried below the left clavicle. There is no particular reason why the pacemaker should be related to the stroke, except that patients with vascular disease in one territory usually have it in others – this man probably has both coronary and cerebrovascular disease.

SUMMARY

Permanent pacemaker and underlying complete block.

 See *ECG Made Easy*, 9th edition, Chapter 8

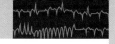

ECG 31

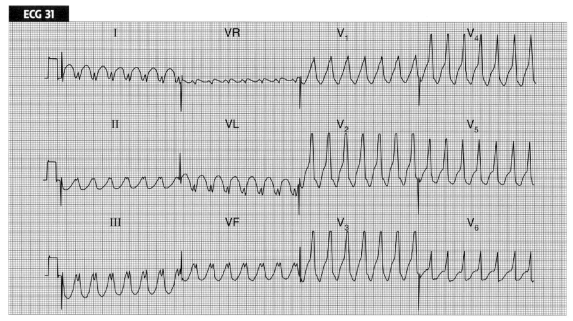

A 60-year-old man complained of severe central chest pain, and a few minutes later became extremely breathless and collapsed. He was brought to the A&E department, where his heart rate was found to be 165 bpm, his blood pressure was unrecordable and he had signs of left ventricular failure. This is his ECG. What has happened and what would you do?

ANSWER 31

The ECG shows:
- Broad complex tachycardia at 165 bpm
- No P waves visible
- QRS complex duration about 200 ms
- Concordance of QRS complexes (i.e. all point upwards) in the chest leads

Clinical interpretation

A broad complex tachycardia can be ventricular in origin, or can be due to a supraventricular tachycardia with aberrant conduction (i.e. bundle branch block). Here the very broad complexes and the QRS complex concordance suggest a ventricular tachycardia. In a patient with a myocardial infarction it is always safe to assume that such a rhythm is ventricular. From the story, one would guess that this patient had a myocardial infarction and then developed ventricular tachycardia, but it is possible that the chest pain was due to the arrhythmia.

What to do

This patient has haemodynamic compromise – low blood pressure and heart failure – and needs immediate cardioversion. An anaesthetic will be required. Following restoration of a less malignant heart rhythm, he is likely to require emergency coronary revascularization with primary angioplasty.

SUMMARY

Ventricular tachycardia.

 See *ECG Made Easy*, 9th edition, Chapter 3

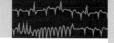

ECG 32

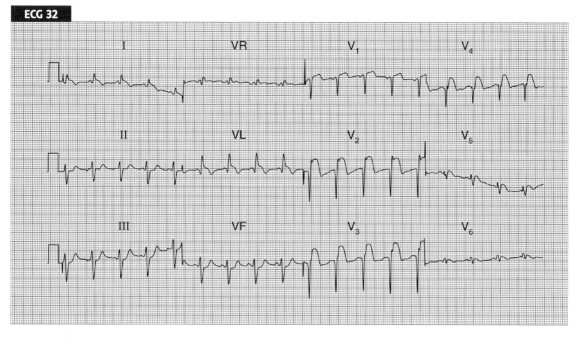

A 45-year-old patient is admitted to the A&E department having had severe central chest pain for 1 h. There are no signs of heart failure, and this is his ECG. What does the ECG show and what would you do?

ANSWER 32

The ECG shows:

- Sinus rhythm, rate 100 bpm
- Left axis deviation
- Q waves in leads V_2–V_4
- Raised ST segments in leads I, VL, V_2–V_5.

Clinical interpretation

This ECG shows left anterior hemiblock, with an acute ST segment elevation anterolateral myocardial infarction (STEMI).

What to do

This patient requires emergency treatment for STEMI. Analgesia, dual antiplatelet therapy (aspirin and P2Y12 inhibitor) and urgent primary percutaneous coronary intervention (PCI) are indicated. Following revascularization secondary prevention therapies should be initiated.

SUMMARY

Acute anterolateral STEMI and left anterior hemiblock.

 See *ECG Made Easy*, 9th edition, Chapter 7

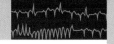

ECG 33

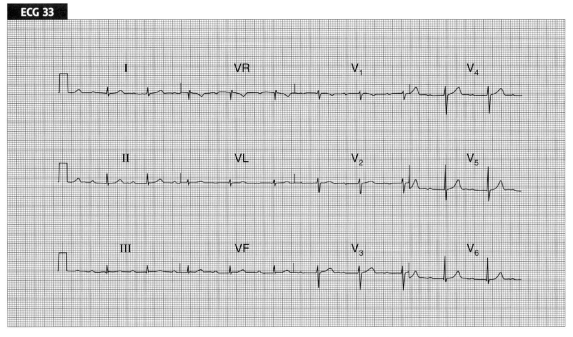

This ECG was recorded from an asymptomatic 45-year-old man at a 'health screening' examination. Is it normal, and what advice would you give him?

ANSWER 33

The ECG shows:

- Sinus rhythm, rate 64 bpm
- Prolonged PR interval (360 ms)
- Normal QRS complexes, ST segments and T waves.

Clinical interpretation

This ECG shows first degree atrioventricular block but is otherwise entirely normal.

What to do

Although the upper limit of the PR interval is usually taken to be 220 ms, longer durations (technically first degree block) are frequently seen in healthy people. Provided you can be sure that this patient has no symptoms, and provided the physical examination is normal, no further action is required. Some individuals in occupations that require a totally normal ECG may have to have an ambulatory ECG recording to demonstrate that there are no episodes of higher-degree block.

SUMMARY

First degree atrioventricular block.

 See *ECG Made Easy*, 9th edition, Chapter 3

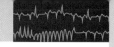

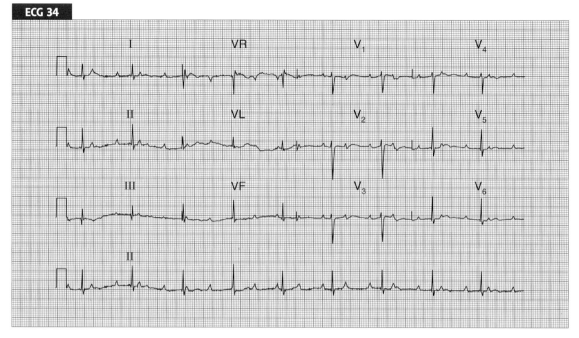

This ECG was recorded from a 70-year-old woman who had complained of attacks of dizziness for about a year. What is the problem, what might be its cause, and how should this woman be treated?

ANSWER 34

The ECG shows:
- Sinus rhythm with complete (third degree) block, rate 55 bpm
- Normal axis
- Normal QRS complexes and T waves.

Clinical interpretation

This ECG shows complete heart block with a relatively low ventricular rate. The attacks of dizziness may be due to further slowing of the heart rate. Although at times there appears to be second degree (2:1) block, the lead II rhythm strip shows that what could be the PR interval is continually changing, and that there is actually no relationship between the P waves and QRS complexes. The QRS complex is narrow, and so must originate in the His bundle.

What to do

The patient needs a permanent pacemaker. There are many causes of heart block, including ischaemia; association with aortic valve calcification; Lyme disease (*Borrelia burgdorferi*); His bundle interruption (due to surgery, trauma, parasites, tumours, abscesses, granulomata); and drugs (digoxin, beta-blockers, calcium-channel blockers). However, most cases of heart block are due to His bundle fibrosis, for which hypertension is a risk factor. An echocardiogram should be arranged to exclude structural heart disease.

SUMMARY

Complete (third degree) block.

 See *ECG Made Easy*, 9th edition, Chapter 3

ECG 35

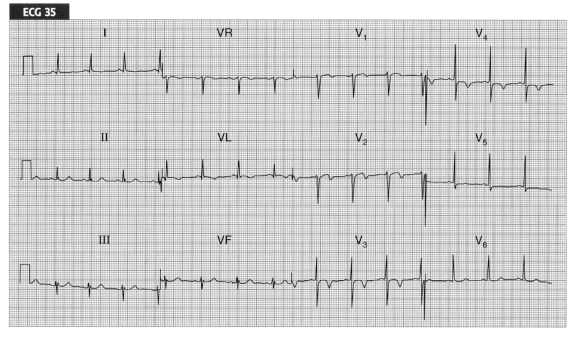

This ECG was recorded in the A&E department from a 60-year-old man who had had intermittent central chest pain for 24 h. What does it show and how should he be managed?

ANSWER 35

The ECG shows:

- Sinus rhythm, rate 81 bpm
- Normal conduction intervals
- Normal axis
- Normal QRS complexes
- Normal ST segments, with ST segment depression in lead V$_4$
- T wave inversion in leads VL, V$_2$–V$_4$.

Clinical interpretation

This ECG shows an anterior non-ST segment elevation myocardial infarction (NSTEMI).

What to do

This patient clearly has an acute coronary syndrome. This will be confirmed by measurement of high sensitivity troponin. He must be admitted to hospital and treated with dual antiplatelet therapy (aspirin and P2Y12 inhibitors) and low-molecular-weight heparin, pending inpatient percutaneous coronary intervention (PCI). Secondary prevention therapies should also be initiated during his admission.

SUMMARY

Anterior NSTEMI.

 See *ECG Made Easy*, 9th edition, Chapter 7

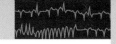

ECG 36

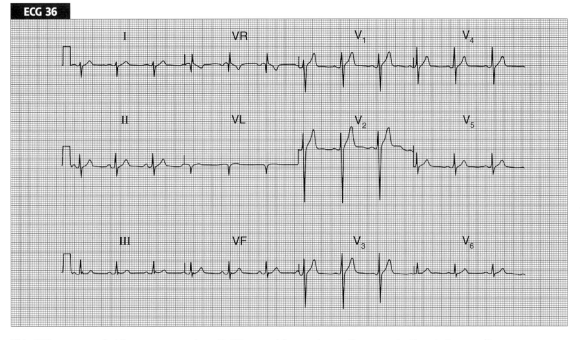

This ECG was recorded from an asymptomatic 30-year-old man at a routine examination. Is it normal?

ANSWER 36

The ECG shows:
- Sinus rhythm, rate 73 bpm
- Right axis deviation (S wave bigger than R wave in lead I, large R wave in lead VR, very small R wave and deep S wave in lead VL)
- Notched QRS complexes in lead III
- Otherwise entirely normal QRS complexes and T waves.

Clinical interpretation

Right axis deviation can be a feature of right ventricular hypertrophy, but in tall, thin people it is a normal variant. The notched QRS complexes in lead III are normal, although if present in all leads and in a different clinical context, they could be the 'J' waves of hypothermia.

What to do

Examine the patient and exclude right ventricular hypertrophy (you should have done this before recording the ECG!) and consider echocardiography if unsure but this ECG is probably normal.

SUMMARY

Normal ECG with right axis deviation.

 See *ECG Made Easy*, 9th edition, Chapter 2

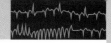

ECG 37

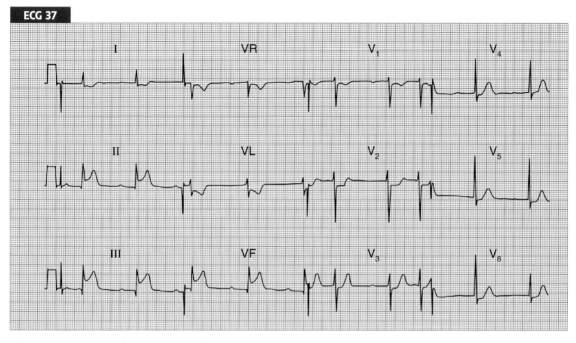

This ECG was recorded from a 55-year-old man who was admitted to hospital as an emergency with severe central chest pain that had been present for about an hour. He was pale, cold and clammy; his blood pressure was 100/80, but there were no signs of heart failure. What does this ECG show? Does anything about it surprise you?

ANSWER 37

The ECG shows:

- Sinus rhythm, rate 50 bpm
- First degree block (PR interval 350 ms)
- Normal axis
- Small Q waves in leads II, III, VF
- Raised ST segments in leads II, III, VF
- Depressed ST segments and inverted T waves in leads I, VL
- Slight ST segment depression in the chest leads.

Clinical interpretation

Acute inferior ST segment elevation myocardial infarction (STEMI) with anterolateral ischaemia, and first degree block. Patients who are in pain with an acute myocardial infarction usually have a sinus tachycardia, but here vagal overactivity is causing a bradycardia.

What to do

This patient should be treated as a STEMI emergency. Analgesia should be administered as required along with dual antiplatelet therapy (aspirin and P2Y12 inhibitor) in preparation for primary percutaneous coronary intervention (PCI). The first degree block does not require specific treatment nor does the relative bradycardia unless this deteriorates further.

SUMMARY

Acute inferior STEMI with first degree block.

 See *ECG Made Easy*, 9th edition, Chapter 7

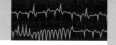

ECG 38

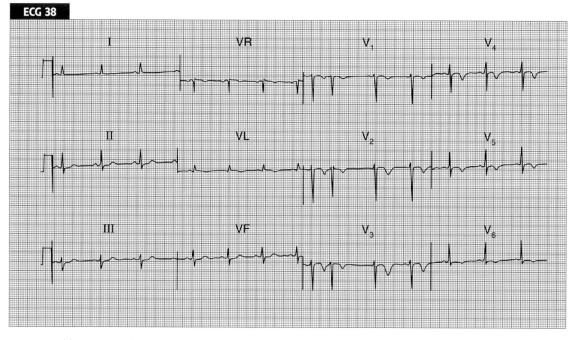

A 50-year-old man was admitted to hospital as an emergency, having had central chest pain for 1 h. By the time he was seen in the A&E department he was pain-free and there were no abnormalities on examination. This is his ECG. What does it show, and what would you do?

ANSWER 38

The ECG shows:
- Sinus rhythm, average rate 75 bpm, with one supraventricular extrasystole; there appears to be an abnormal P wave in lead V_1, so the extrasystole is atrial in origin
- Normal axis
- Normal QRS complexes
- Inverted T waves in leads VL, V_1–V_6.

Clinical interpretation

There are many causes of inverted T waves, and ECGs should always be interpreted as part of the overall clinical picture. In this case the history suggests a myocardial infarction, and the ECG is characteristic of an acute anterior non-ST segment elevation myocardial infarction (NSTEMI).

What to do

Although the patient is now asymptomatic he should remain in hospital for observation and measurement of high sensitivity troponin. He should be started on dual antiplatelet therapy (aspirin and P2Y12 inhibitor) and an anticoagulant (e.g. low molecular weight heparin or fondaparinux) pending coronary angiography. He will also require optimal secondary prevention therapies.

SUMMARY

Anterolateral NSTEMI.

 See *ECG Made Easy*, 9th edition, Chapter 7

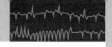

ECG 39

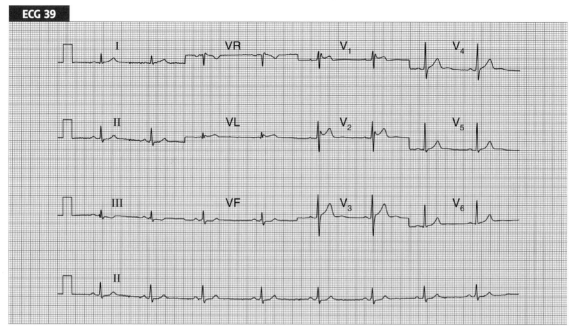

This ECG was recorded as part of the routine preoperative assessment of a 65-year-old man who had no cardiovascular symptoms, and whose heart was clinically normal. What does it show? Is any action necessary?

ANSWER 39

The ECG shows:
- Sinus rhythm, rate 50 bpm
- Normal axis
- QRS complex duration 110 ms, with an RSR^1 pattern in leads V$_1$ and V$_2$ – partial right bundle branch block (RBBB).

Clinical interpretation

The QRS complex duration is at the upper limit of normal, so this is partial rather than complete RBBB. It is seldom of any clinical significance.

What to do

In the absence of symptoms or abnormal signs, no action is necessary.

SUMMARY

Partial RBBB.

 See *ECG Made Easy*, 9th edition, Chapter 6

ECG 40

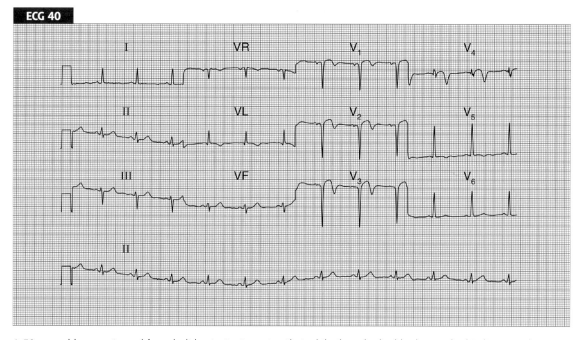

A 50-year-old man returned from holiday in Spain saying that while there he had had some bad indigestion, but was now perfectly well. This is his ECG: what does it show and what would you do?

ANSWER 40

The ECG shows:
- Sinus rhythm, rate 72 bpm
- Normal conduction
- Normal axis
- Q waves in leads V_2–V_3
- Elevated ST segments in leads V_2–V_4
- Inverted T waves in leads VL, V_1–V_5.

Clinical interpretation

This ECG shows an old anterior myocardial infarction. The elevation of ST segments might suggest an acute process if the pain were recent, but with this story the changes are almost certainly old. The persistence of ST segment elevation in the anterior leads may be due to a left ventricular aneurysm.

What to do

The assumption has to be that the 'indigestion' was actually a myocardial infarction. Since he is now well, the important thing is to ensure that he takes the appropriate steps to prevent a further attack – he must stop smoking and reduce weight if necessary, and he should be treated with dual antiplatelet therapy (aspirin and a P2Y12 inhibitor), a beta-blocker, an angiotensin-converting enzyme inhibitor and a statin in accordance with guidelines. His coronary disease will require further investigation, probably with coronary angiography, although a cardiac stress MRI may be helpful first to determine the extent of left ventricular impairment (and infarction) as well as any residual areas of ischaemia and viability.

> **SUMMARY**
>
> Old anterior myocardial infarction.

 See *ECG Made Easy*, 9th edition, Chapter 7

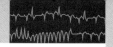

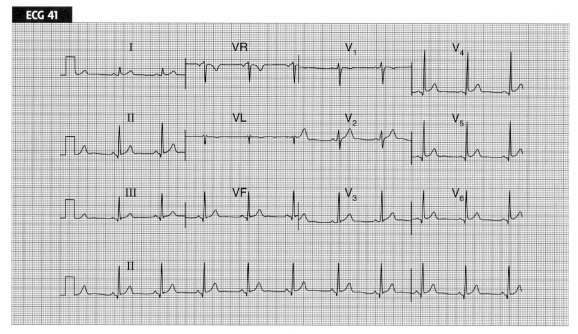

This ECG was recorded from a 30-year-old man who complained of chest pain: the pain did not appear to be cardiac in origin, and the physical examination was normal. Can this man be allowed to hold a commercial driving licence?

ANSWER 41

The ECG shows:

- Sinus rhythm, rate 62 bpm
- Normal axis
- Small Q waves, especially prominent in leads II, III, VF, V_4–V_6
- Otherwise normal QRS complexes, ST segments and T waves.

Clinical interpretation

These Q waves are quite deep but only 40 ms in duration, and they are most prominent in the lateral leads. They represent septal depolarization, not an old lateral infarction.

What to do

The ECG is normal, and if the man has no other evidence of heart disease he can hold a commercial driving licence. If in doubt, a coronary CT scan should be confirmatory.

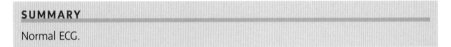

SUMMARY

Normal ECG.

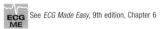 See *ECG Made Easy*, 9th edition, Chapter 6

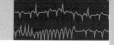

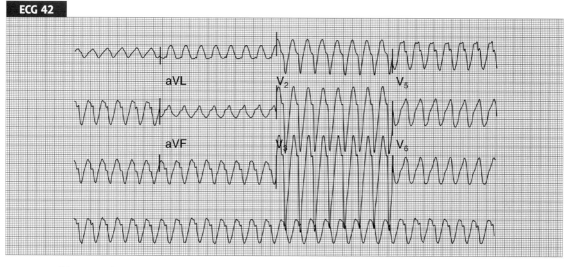

A 45-year-old man in the Coronary Care Unit with a suspected myocardial infarction suddenly becomes breathless and hypotensive, and this is his ECG. What does it show and what would you do?

ANSWER 42

This ECG shows:
- A broad complex tachycardia
- Heart rate 180 bpm
- No P waves visible
- QRS duration about 200 ms
- It is difficult to be sure whether the complexes are pointing upwards or downwards, but the axis appears to be to the left.

Clinical interpretation

A broad complex tachycardia can in theory be due either to a supraventricular tachycardia with bundle branch block, or to ventricular tachycardia. The very broad complexes with left axis deviation suggest that this is ventricular tachycardia. More important, however, is the clinical context: in a patient with a suspected myocardial infarction with a first attack of tachycardia, a broad complex rhythm is almost certainly ventricular tachycardia.

What to do

Since the patient is breathless with a low blood pressure, immediate cardioversion under sedation of anaesthesia is indicated. Once a safe rhythm has been restored, attention should be turned to management of his myocardial infarction, including emergency coronary angiography and percutaneous intervention.

> **SUMMARY**
>
> Ventricular tachycardia.

 See *ECG Made Easy*, 9th edition, Chapter 8

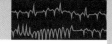
ECG 43

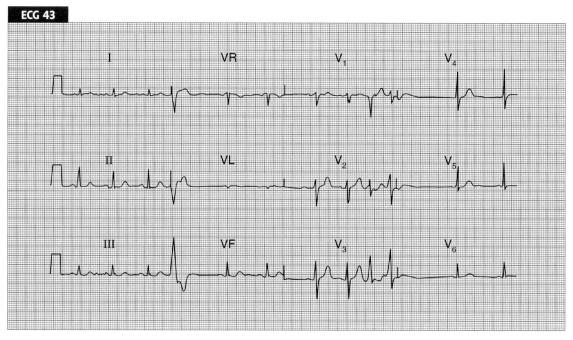

This ECG was recorded from an 80-year-old man during a routine preoperative assessment. What does it show? What are the implications for surgery?

ANSWER 43

The ECG shows:
- Sinus rhythm, rate about 77 bpm, with ventricular extrasystoles
- Ventricular extrasystoles are of two types, seen best in lead V_3
- Normal axis
- Normal QRS complexes in the sinus beats
- ST segments and T waves are normal in the sinus beats.

Clinical interpretation

Sinus rhythm, with multifocal ventricular extrasystoles but otherwise normal.

What to do

In large groups of patients, ventricular extrasystoles are correlated with heart disease of all types. In individuals, however, extrasystoles may well occur in a perfectly normal heart – indeed, virtually everyone has extrasystoles at times. Ventricular extrasystoles become more common with increasing age, and this patient is 80 years old. In the absence of symptoms or clinical signs suggesting cardiovascular disease, the extrasystoles probably do not have any great significance. Echocardiography to confirm a structurally normal heart with normal systolic function will provide further reassurance of the patient's cardiovascular fitness for surgery. The ventricular extrasystoles do not require specific treatment.

SUMMARY

Sinus rhythm with multifocal ventricular extrasystoles.

 See *ECG Made Easy*, 9th edition, Chapter 4

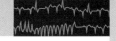

ECG 44

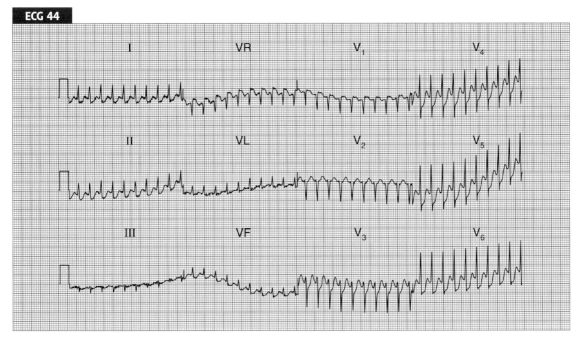

A 50-year-old man was admitted to hospital as an emergency with chest pain; he was not aware of a rapid heart rate. He had had several episodes of pain that appeared to be due to ischaemia, but they had no clear relationship with exertion. Shortly after this ECG was recorded, his heart rate suddenly slowed and his ECG was then normal. What does this record show, and what would you do?

ANSWER 44

The ECG shows:
- Narrow complex tachycardia, rate about 230 bpm
- No P waves
- Normal axis
- Normal QRS complexes
- Horizontal ST segment depression, most marked in leads V$_4$–V$_6$.

Clinical interpretation

Narrow complex tachycardia without P waves – atrioventricular nodal re-entry (junctional) tachycardia (AVNRT) or atrioventricular re-entry tachycardia (AVRT). Ischaemic ST segment depression, accounting for his pain.

What to do

Not all patients with a paroxysmal tachycardia complain of palpitations; this patient's recurrent chest pain may well have been due to this arrhythmia. Prophylactic drug therapy will be needed: a beta-blocker or verapamil should be tried first. Electrophysiological investigation, with a view to ablating an abnormal pathway, may be needed.

SUMMARY

Atrioventricular nodal re-entry (junctional) tachycardia (AVNRT) with ischaemia.

 See *ECG Made Easy*, 9th edition, Chapter 4

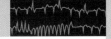

ECG 45

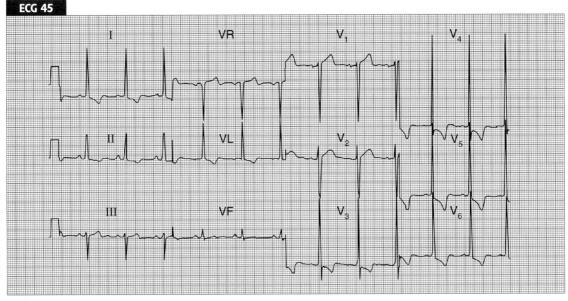

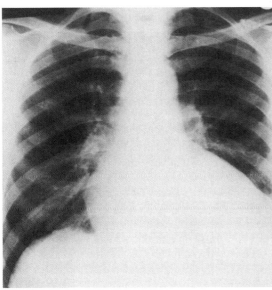

An 85-year-old man, who has had high blood pressure for many years, is seen in the outpatient department complaining of typical angina and of occasional dizziness when walking up hills. These are his ECG and chest X-ray. What is the diagnosis, and what would you do?

ANSWER 45

The ECG shows:
- Sinus rhythm, rate 71 bpm
- Normal axis
- Tall R waves and deep S waves in the chest leads
- ST segment depression in leads V_4–V_6
- Inverted T waves in leads I, II, VL, V_3–V_6.

The chest X-ray shows a large heart, due to left ventricular hypertrophy.

Clinical interpretation

This is marked left ventricular hypertrophy. It can be difficult to distinguish between T wave inversion due to ischaemia and the T wave inversion of left ventricular hypertrophy, and when the T wave is inverted in the septal leads (V_3–V_4), ischaemia has to be considered. However, here the change is most marked in the lateral leads, and is associated with the 'voltage criteria' for left ventricular hypertrophy. Angina, dizziness and left ventricular hypertrophy in an 85-year-old may be due to tight aortic stenosis, although hypertension is a possibility.

What to do

Look for the signs of aortic stenosis ('plateau' pulse, narrow pulse pressure, displaced apex beat, aortic ejection systolic murmur) and confirm the valve gradient with echocardiography. In this patient the aortic valve gradient was 20 mmHg, indicating trivial stenosis of the valve, so the left ventricular hypertrophy is most likely to be due to the long-standing hypertension. The angina may well improve with adequate blood pressure control and the usual anti-anginal medication, but if it does not, then coronary angiography with a view to percutaneous coronary intervention (PCI) or bypass surgery should be considered.

SUMMARY

Left ventricular hypertrophy.

 See *ECG Made Easy*, 9th edition, Chapter 5

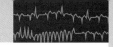

ECG 46

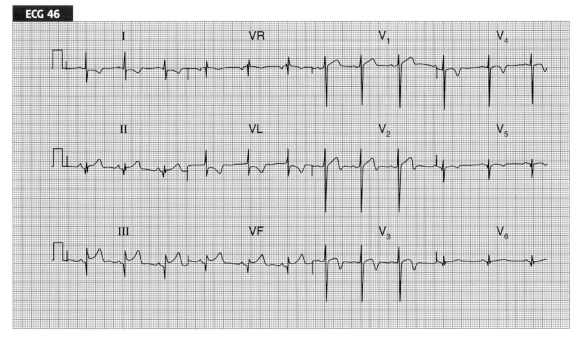

A 70-year-old man, who has had angina for 10 years, is admitted to hospital with severe central chest pain that has been present for 4 h. This is his ECG. What does it show, and what would you do?

ANSWER 46

The ECG shows:
- Sinus rhythm, average rate 70 bpm
- Normal axis
- Q waves in leads III, VF
- Normal QRS complexes elsewhere
- Raised ST segments in leads II (following small S waves), III, VF
- Biphasic T waves in leads V_2–V_3
- Inverted T waves in leads V_4–V_5.

Clinical interpretation

The inferior Q waves suggest an old infarction. The raised ST segments in leads III and VF would be compatible with an acute infarction, though the raised ST segment in lead II is a 'high take-off' segment because it follows an S wave, and this raises the possibility that the changes in leads III and VF may not be significant. The anterior changes suggest a non-ST segment elevation myocardial infarction (NSTEMI). Taken together with his presentation, this is a high-risk ECG.

What to do

There is enough evidence here to justify urgent management as a STEMI. The patient should be treated with analgesia as required, dual antiplatelet therapy (with aspirin and a P2Y12 inhibitor) and primary percutaneous coronary intervention (PCI). Optimal secondary prevention therapies will be required after revascularization.

SUMMARY

Possible old and/or possible new inferior myocardial infarction; anterior NSTEMI. High risk acute coronary syndrome.

 See *ECG Made Easy*, 9th edition, Chapter 7

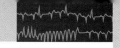

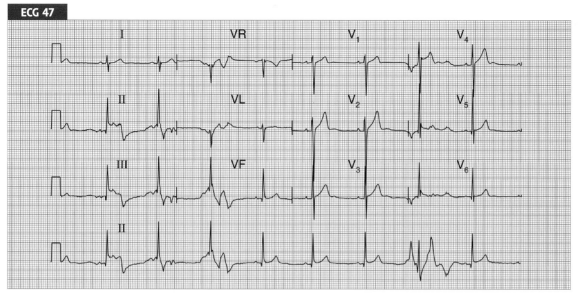

This was a routine ECG recorded pre-operatively in a 60-year-old woman due for a cholecystectomy. Can the operation go ahead?

ANSWER 47

This ECG shows:
- Three complexes in the middle of the record which are clearly sinus rhythm
- Rate 57 bpm
- Remaining complexes are a bizarre and variable shape and the T waves cannot be identified, but these complexes are at the same rate as those in sinus rhythm.

Clinical interpretation

At first sight the abnormal complexes might be ventricular extrasystoles, but this is very unlikely because they are such an abnormal shape and have no obvious T waves. More importantly, they occur at the time that would be expected if the rhythm was sinus rhythm throughout. These complexes must be artefacts, due to poor electrode contact with the skin.

What to do

Although all the beats that clearly show sinus rhythm are normal, the ECG is incomplete and must be repeated.

> **SUMMARY**
>
> Artefacts due to poor electrode contact.

 See *ECG Made Easy*, 9th edition, Chapter 2

ECG 48

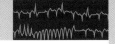

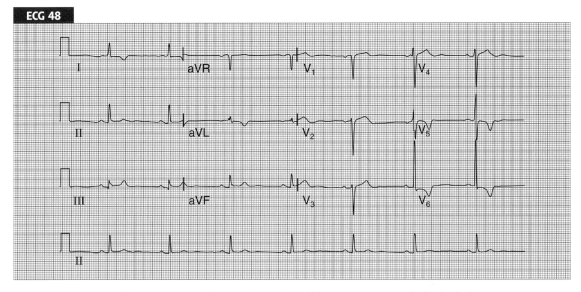

This ECG was recorded from a 50-year-old man who was breathless on exertion and who had a heart murmur. Are the changes significant?

ANSWER 48

This ECG shows:
- Sinus rhythm at 45 bpm
- Normal axis
- Left ventricular hypertrophy on voltage criteria (R wave in V_6=35 mm)
- Inverted T waves in leads 1, VL, V_5 and V_6.

Clinical interpretation

This is the classical ECG appearance of left ventricular hypertrophy. Since he has a heart murmur, the most likely diagnosis is aortic stenosis. The differential diagnosis includes hypertrophic obstructive cardiomyopathy.

What to do

A patient who is breathless, has a heart murmur and who has marked left ventricular hypertrophy on the ECG needs an urgent echocardiogram. This patient had severe aortic stenosis and needed an aortic valve replacement.

> **SUMMARY**
>
> Left ventricular hypertrophy.

 See *ECG Made Easy*, 9th edition, Chapter 5

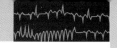

ECG 49

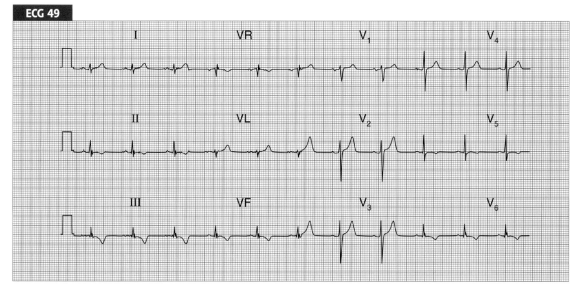

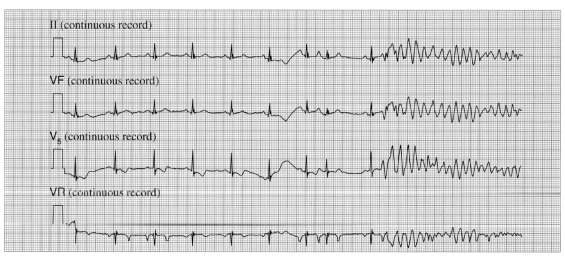

A 50-year-old man, who had had exertional chest pain for some months, was seen in the A&E department with persistent central chest pain which had commenced 1 h earlier. These are his ECGs. What does the upper ECG show and what would you do? The lower ECG shows what happened when an exercise test was performed.

ANSWER 49

The top ECG shows:
- Sinus rhythm, rate 65 bpm
- Normal axis
- 'Splintered' QRS complex in leads II,III, VF, V$_6$ – otherwise normal QRS complexes, duration 100 ms
- T waves inverted in leads II–III, VF, V$_5$–V$_6$.

Clinical interpretation

The 'splintered' QRS complex in the inferior leads is probably of no significance. The T wave inversion in the inferior and lateral leads suggests a non-ST segment elevation myocardial infarction (NSTEMI).

What to do

This patient clearly has an acute coronary syndrome. This will be confirmed by measurement of high sensitivity troponin. Following analgesia if needed, he should be loaded with dual antiplatelet therapy (aspirin and a P2Y12 inhibitor). He will require coronary angiography with a view to coronary revascularization (percutaneous coronary intervention [PCI] or coronary artery bypass graft [CABG]). If his symptoms do not settle with initial medical therapies (e.g. a beta-blocker and nitrates [intravenous or buccal]), this should be arranged urgently. Otherwise it should be arranged in the next 48 hours. During the initial treatment phase, the ECG should be recorded every half-hour to see if ST segment elevation appears.

Exercise testing would no-longer be guideline-based treatment for this presentation. However in this historical case, an exercise test was conducted to try to determine prioritization for inpatient angiography.

Exercise test

The lower ECG, recorded in stage 2 of the Bruce protocol, after 4 min and 41 s, shows:
- Sudden onset of ventricular fibrillation.

What to do

Immediate resuscitation in accordance with ALS guidelines. Exercise testing is no longer recommended as part of the assessment of patients with acute coronary syndromes.

SUMMARY

Inferolateral NSTEMI; ventricular fibrillation during exercise testing.

ECG ME   See *ECG Made Easy*, 9th edition, Chapter 4

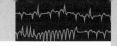
ECG 50

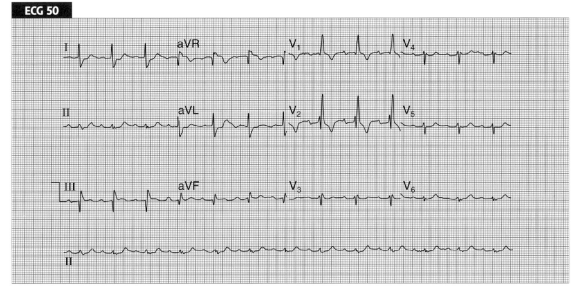

This ECG was recorded from a 60-year-old man who had had an episode of chest pain a year previously, and now complained of breathlessness and occasional dizziness.

ANSWER 50

This ECG shows:
- Sinus rhythm, rate 80 bpm
- First degree block – PR interval 250 ms
- Right bundle branch block (RBBB)
- Q waves in leads III and VF.

Clinical interpretation

The Q waves in the inferior leads suggest an old myocardial infarction, which would fit with his history of chest pain. Without a previous ECG it is difficult to know whether the RBBB is new or old, but the combination of RBBB and first degree block raises the possibility that his dizziness is due to intermittent complete block.

What to do

He needs investigations to assess the extent of LV dysfunction, evaluate his coronary artery disease and to exclude arrhythmia as a cause for his dizziness. A cardiac stress MRI will determine LV function, the extent of infarction versus viability and the ischaemic burden. Ambulatory ECG recording will be required to investigate the dizziness, in the first instance with a 24 hour tape recording.

SUMMARY

First degree block and RBBB.

 See *ECG Made Easy*, 9th edition, Chapter 3

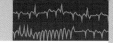

ECG 51

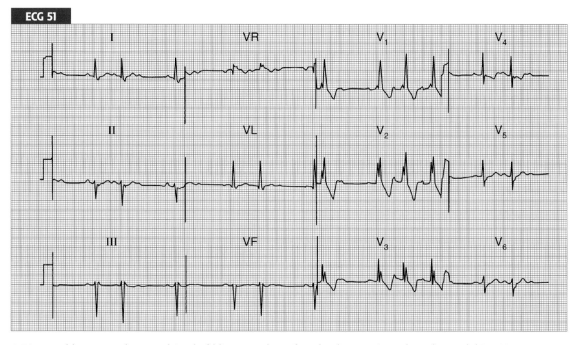

A 70-year-old woman who complained of 'dizzy turns' was found to have an irregular pulse, and this ECG was recorded. There are three abnormalities. What advice would you give her?

ANSWER 51

The ECG shows:
- Sinus rhythm; sinus rate 100 bpm
- Normal and constant PR intervals in the conducted beats
- Occasional nonconducted P waves (best seen in lead I)
- Left axis deviation
- Right bundle branch block (RBBB).

Clinical interpretation

This ECG shows second degree block (Mobitz type 2) and bifascicular block – left axis deviation (left anterior hemiblock) and RBBB. This combination of conduction abnormalities indicates disease throughout the conduction system, and is sometimes called 'trifascicular' block.

What to do

The 'dizzy turns' may represent intermittent complete block. Permanent pacing is essential.

SUMMARY

Second degree block (Mobitz type 2) and bifascicular block.

 See *ECG Made Easy*, 9th edition, Chapter 3

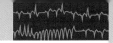

ECG 52

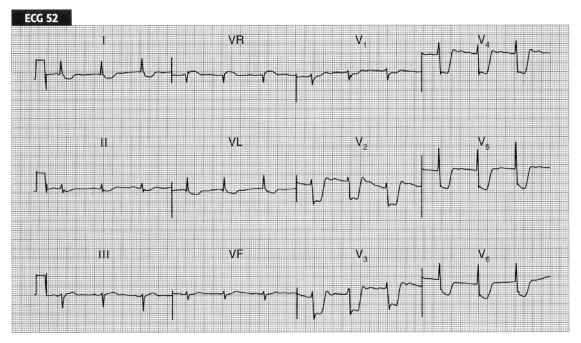

An 80-year-old man being observed in the recovery room following a femoral–popliteal bypass operation was noted to have this abnormal ECG. What does it show and what would you do?

ANSWER 52

The ECG shows:
- Sinus rhythm, rate 68 bpm
- Normal axis
- Normal QRS complexes
- Marked horizontal ST segment depression (about 8 mm) in leads V_2–V_4, and downward-sloping ST segment depression in the lateral leads.

Clinical interpretation

The patient is elderly and has peripheral vascular disease, so coronary disease is likely to be present. The appearance of the ECG is characteristic of severe cardiac ischaemia. The lack of a tachycardia is surprising.

What to do

This is not an easy situation to deal with because the patient's postoperative condition dictates management. This requires careful multidisciplinary management in a high-dependency area. Oxygen therapy should be given for low saturations and significant anaemia corrected. Ideally he needs dual antiplatelet therapy and anticoagulation, though his postoperative state may prevent this. If blood pressure allows, intravenous nitrates should be given cautiously. Coronary intervention (via a radial approach) in this context would be high risk.

SUMMARY

Severe anterolateral ischaemia.

 See *ECG Made Easy*, 9th edition, Chapter 7

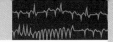

ECG 53

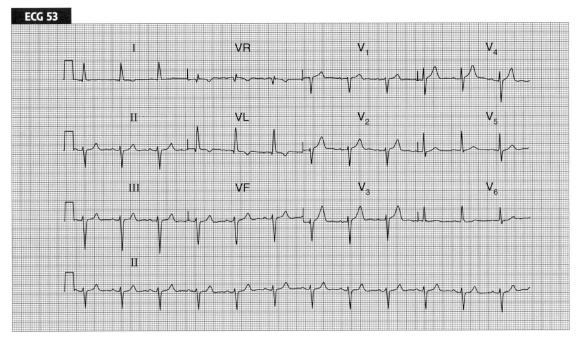

A 70-year-old man had had high blood pressure for many years, but it was now well controlled at 140/85. He had no symptoms, and no abnormalities were detected on physical examination. This ECG was recorded during a routine follow-up appointment. Does it give any cause for concern, and if so, what would you do?

ANSWER 53

The ECG shows:
- Sinus rhythm, rate 73 bpm
- Normal PR interval
- Left axis deviation (left anterior hemiblock)
- Normal QRS complexes
- T wave inversion in leads I and VL.

Clinical interpretation

The left axis deviation indicates a conduction defect in the anterior fascicle of the left bundle branch – left anterior hemiblock. This is due to fibrosis, almost certainly the result of long-standing hypertension. The T wave inversion in the lateral leads (I and VL) probably indicates left ventricular hypertrophy, although the QRS complex in lead V_6 is not unusually tall and the 'voltage criteria' for left ventricular hypertrophy are not met.

What to do

This man clearly has 'target organ' (heart) damage as the result of his hypertension. An echocardiogram should be recorded to assess his left ventricular thickness and function, because the prognosis is worse if there is left ventricular hypertrophy or if there is any reduction in function. The presence of other risk factors, such as diabetes and hypercholesterolaemia, must be checked and, if necessary, treated. If there is any suggestion of angina, further investigation may be merited, but if he really is completely asymptomatic this is probably not essential. Careful control of his blood pressure is the key to management.

SUMMARY

Left anterior hemiblock and either left ventricular hypertrophy.

 See *ECG Made Easy*, 9th edition, Chapter 3

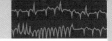

ECG 54

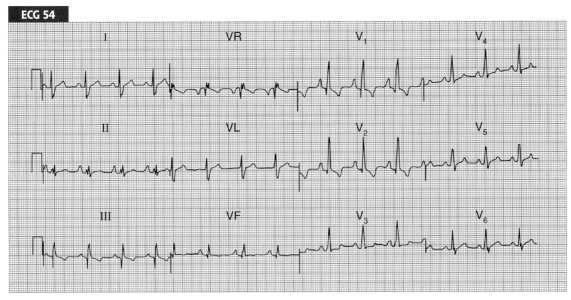

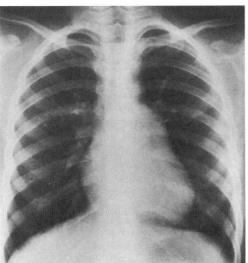

This ECG and chest X-ray were recorded from a 17-year-old girl who was breathless, had marked ankle swelling with signs of right heart failure, and who had been known to have a heart murmur since birth. She was acyanotic. What ECG abnormalities can you identify, and can you suggest a diagnosis?

ANSWER 54

The ECG shows:
- Sinus rhythm, rate 81 bpm
- Markedly peaked P waves (best seen in leads II, V$_1$)
- Normal axis
- Dominant R wave in lead V$_1$.

The chest X-ray shows a high and prominent cardiac apex, consistent with right ventricular hypertrophy, and a prominent pulmonary artery (arrowed) which is due to post-stenotic dilatation as a result of pulmonary stenosis.

Clinical interpretation

The ECG shows right atrial and right ventricular hypertrophy.

What to do

Right atrial hypertrophy is seen with pulmonary hypertension of any cause, tricuspid stenosis and Ebstein's anomaly. Right ventricular hypertrophy is seen with pulmonary stenosis and pulmonary hypertension. These conditions can all be diagnosed by echocardiography. This patient had pulmonary stenosis.

SUMMARY

Right atrial and right ventricular hypertrophy.

 See *ECG Made Easy*, 9th edition, Chapter 5

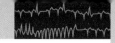

ECG 55

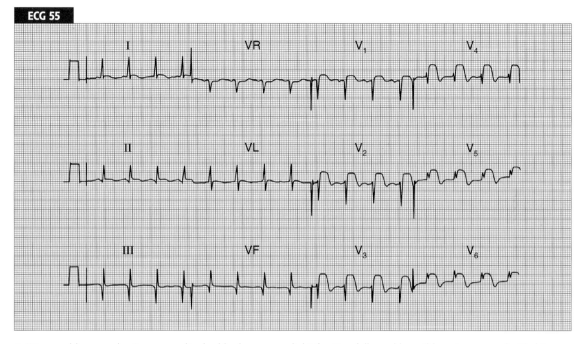

A 60-year-old man, who 3 years earlier had had a myocardial infarction followed by mild angina, was admitted to hospital with central chest pain that had been present for 1 h and had not responded to sublingual nitrates. What does his ECG show, and what would you do?

ANSWER 55

The ECG shows:
- Sinus rhythm, rate 103 bpm
- Normal axis
- Q waves in leads II, III, VF
- Normal QRS complexes in the anterior leads
- Marked ST segment elevation in leads V_1–V_6.

Clinical interpretation

The Q waves in leads III and VF suggest an old inferior infarction, while the elevated ST segments in leads V_1–V_6 indicate an acute anterior ST segment elevation infarction (STEMI).

What to do

The patient should be given pain relief as required and initiated on dual antiplatelet therapy (with aspirin and a P2Y12 inhibitor) followed by immediate primary percutaneous coronary intervention (PCI). Secondary prevention therapies should be initiated following revascularization.

SUMMARY

Old inferior and acute anterior STEMI.

 See *ECG Made Easy*, 9th edition, Chapter 7

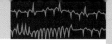

ECG 56

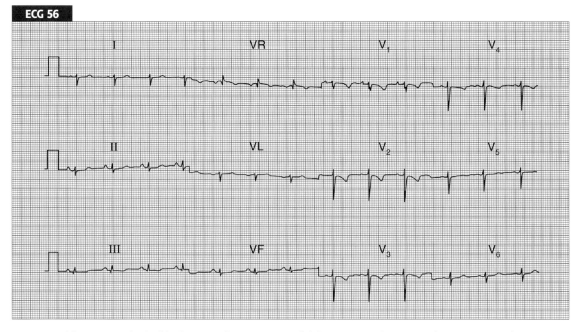

A 32-year-old woman, who had had a normal pregnancy and delivery 3 months previously, was seen in the outpatient department complaining of severe breathlessness and dizziness on exertion. She had some chest pain on both sides, which sounded pleuritic. Does her ECG help with her diagnosis and treatment?

ANSWER 56

The ECG shows:

- Sinus rhythm, rate 79 bpm
- Right axis deviation
- Normal QRS complexes, except for an RSR^1 pattern in lead V_1 and deep S waves in lead V_6
- Inverted T waves in leads V_1–V_4.

Clinical interpretation

The right axis deviation, the deep S waves in lead V_6 ('clockwise rotation') and the inverted T waves in the chest leads are all characteristic of marked right ventricular hypertrophy: the only missing feature is the absence of dominant R waves in lead V_1. Note how the T wave inversion is at a maximum in lead V_1 and becomes progressively less marked from lead V_2 to V_4.

What to do

In the context of a delivery 3 months previously, this ECG pattern of right ventricular hypertrophy almost certainly indicates multiple pulmonary emboli causing pulmonary hypertension. A computed tomography (CT) pulmonary angiogram confirmed this diagnosis. Anticoagulants, and possibly thrombolysis, are needed urgently.

> **SUMMARY**
>
> Right ventricular hypertrophy due to pulmonary embolism.

 See *ECG Made Easy*, 9th edition, Chapter 7

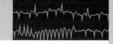

ECG 57

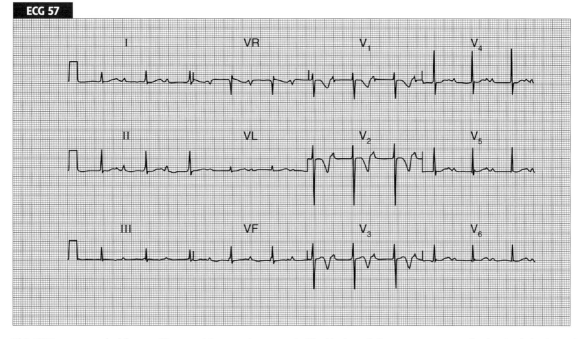

This ECG was recorded from a 50-year-old man who was admitted to hospital as an emergency, having had chest pain characteristic of a myocardial infarction for 3 h. What does the ECG show, and how should the patient be treated?

ANSWER 57

The ECG shows:
- Sinus rhythm, rate 65 bpm
- PR interval markedly prolonged (480 ms)
- Normal axis
- Normal QRS complexes
- T wave inversion in leads V_1–V_3.

Clinical interpretation

First degree block associated with a non-ST segment elevation anterior myocardial infarction (NSTEMI). Since the T wave inversion is in leads V_1–V_3 but not V_4, the possibility of a pulmonary embolus must be considered in the differential diagnosis.

What to do

Echocardiography may show regional wall motion abnormalities in keeping with myocardial infarction and high sensitivity troponin should be measured. The ECG changes do not meet the conventional criteria for primary percutaneous coronary intervention (PCI) (raised ST segments or new left bundle branch block), but the patient does need the full range of treatment for an NSTEMI, which are dual antiplatelet therapy (with aspirin and a P2Y12 inhibitor), anticoagulation (e.g. with low molecular weight heparin or fondaparinux), a nitrate and secondary prevention therapies. Early angiography must be considered with a view to revascularization. If symptoms do not settle or ECG changes deteriorate on close monitoring, this may be required urgently. The first degree block does not require specific treatment and is not a contraindication to betablockade (although ECG monitoring during initiation is sensible).

> **SUMMARY**
>
> First degree block and anterior NSTEMI.

 See *ECG Made Easy*, 9th edition, Chapter 7

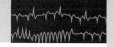

ECG 58

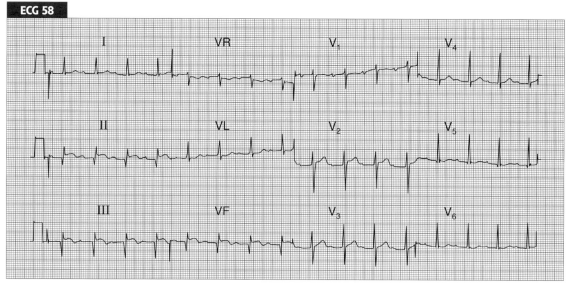

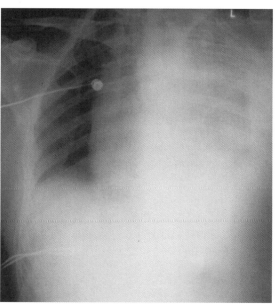

This ECG and chest X-ray were recorded in the A&E department from a 50-year-old man with severe central chest pain that radiated into his back. The pain had been present for 6 h. What do the ECG and X-ray show, and what would you do?

ANSWER 58

The ECG shows:

- Sinus rhythm, rate 88 bpm
- PR interval 320 ms – first degree block
- Q waves in leads II, III, VF
- Raised ST segments in leads II, III, VF
- Inverted T waves in leads III, VF.

The chest X-ray shows opacification of the left side of the chest, with probable shift of the mediastinum to the right.

Clinical interpretation

This ECG shows an acute inferior myocardial infarction, which often causes first degree block. The Q waves and raised ST segments are consistent with the story of 6 h of chest pain, and the first degree block is not important.

What to do

Chest pain radiating through to the back has to raise the possibility of aortic dissection, which can occlude the opening of the coronary arteries and so cause a myocardial infarction. However, it should be noted that this is relatively rare compared with back pain associated with myocardial infarction, which is common. In this case, the chest X-ray suggests that blood has leaked into the left pleural cavity from a dissection of the aorta. The patient needs immediate investigation by computed tomography (CT) or magnetic resonance (MR) scanning and consideration of surgical repair of the dissection. Control of pain and avoidance of hypertension in the interim are important.

> **SUMMARY**
>
> Acute inferior myocardial infarction with first degree block, due to dissection of the aorta.

 See *ECG Made Easy*, 9th edition, Chapter 7

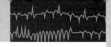

ECG 59

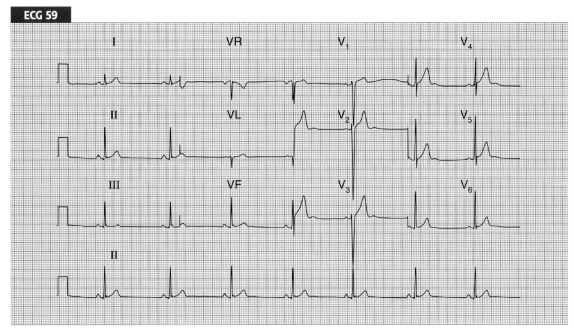

This ECG was recorded from a fit 22-year-old male medical student. He was worried – should he have been?

ANSWER 59

The ECG shows:
- Sinus rhythm, rate 44 bpm
- Normal axis
- Tall R waves (23 mm in lead V_5) and deep S waves (41 mm in lead V_2)
- Normal ST segments and T waves
- Prominent U waves in leads V_2–V_5.

Clinical interpretation

This record shows left ventricular hypertrophy by 'voltage criteria' (R waves greater than 25 mm in lead V_5 or V_6, or the sum of the R wave in lead V_5 or V_6 plus the S wave in lead V_1 or V_2 is greater than 35 mm). There are, however, no T wave changes. 'Voltage criteria' on their own are unreliable, and in a fit young man this may well be a normal variant. The U waves are perfectly normal, and this pattern is common in athletes.

What to do

Tell the student to buy a good book on ECG interpretation, but if reassurance is not enough, echocardiography could be used to measure the left ventricular thickness.

SUMMARY

Left ventricular hypertrophy on 'voltage criteria', but probably normal.

 See *ECG Made Easy*, 9th edition, Chapter 6

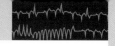

ECG 60

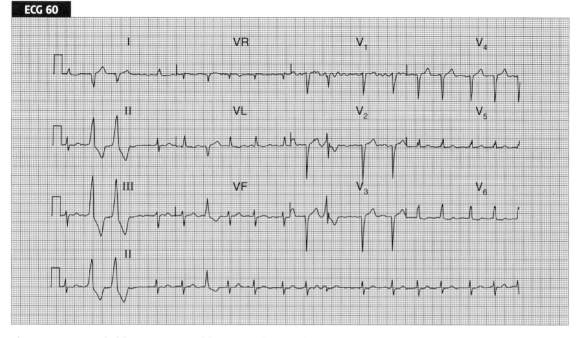

This ECG was recorded from a 70-year-old woman who complained of an irregular heartbeat. What does it show and what would you do?

ANSWER 60

The ECG shows:
- Atrial fibrillation, rate about 110 bpm
- Frequent multifocal ventricular extrasystoles
- Normal axis in the supraventricular beats
- Loss of R waves in leads V_3–V_4
- There is downward-sloping ST segment depression in lead V_6.

Clinical interpretation

This ECG shows an old anterior myocardial infarction, which is probably (but not certainly) the cause of the patient's atrial fibrillation and extrasystoles. The ventricular rate is not well controlled. The ST segment depression may be part of the electrical changes arising from her ischaemic cardiomyopathy or may suggest that she is taking digoxin.

What to do

Remember that in older patients atrial fibrillation may be the only indication of thyrotoxicosis. It would be prudent to check the patient's serum potassium and digoxin levels (if relevant) to make sure that the extrasystoles are not a manifestation of digoxin toxicity. An echocardiogram should be recorded to check her heart size and left ventricular function. Her complaint of palpitations may be due to her atrial fibrillation or to the extrasystoles (or both). A beta-blocker may reduce the extrasystoles as well as control her ventricular rate. Anticoagulation should be considered because of her atrial fibrillation and she may also merit treatment for left ventricular systolic dysfunction and secondary prevention for ischaemic heart disease.

> **SUMMARY**
>
> Atrial fibrillation, multifocal ventricular extrasystoles, and an old anterior myocardial infarction.

 See *ECG Made Easy*, 9th edition, Chapter 4

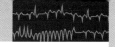

ECG 61

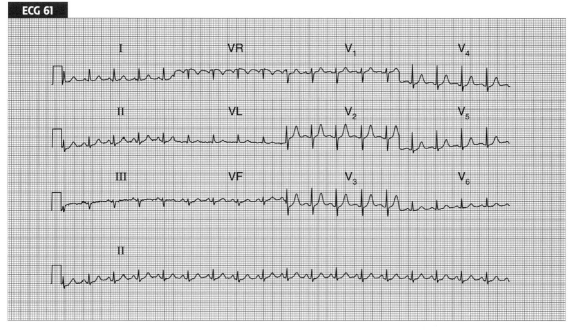

A 45-year-old man complained of palpitations, weight loss and anxiety. His blood pressure was 180/110, and his heart seemed normal. This is his ECG. His thyroid function tests, measured several times, were normal. What might be going on?

ANSWER 61

The ECG shows:
- Narrow complex rhythm at 110 bpm
- One P wave per QRS complex – sinus tachycardia
- Normal PR interval
- Normal axis
- Normal QRS complexes.

Clinical interpretation

The most common causes of a sinus tachycardia are exercise and anxiety, but this patient was losing weight, and although he was anxious it is necessary to think about other diagnoses. His diastolic blood pressure was high, which should not happen with anxiety. He was not thyrotoxic, but there must have been some other physical cause of his problems – it turned out he had a phaeochromocytoma.

SUMMARY

Sinus tachycardia.

 See *ECG Made Easy*, 9th edition, Chapter 6

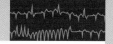

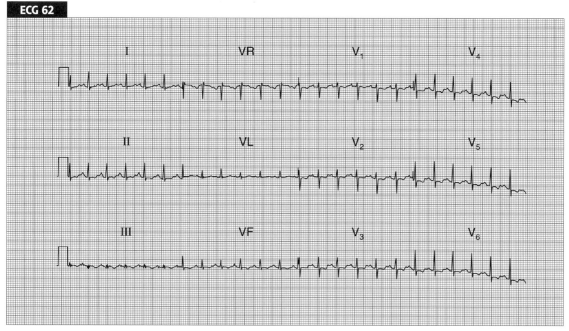

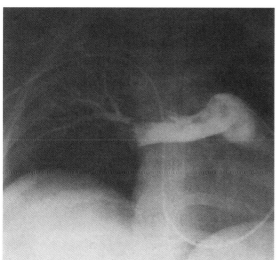

This ECG and pulmonary angiogram are from a 39-year-old woman who complained of a recent sudden onset of breathlessness. She had no previous history of breathlessness, and no chest pain. Examination revealed nothing, other than a rapid heart rate. A pulmonary angiogram was carried out as part of a series of investigations immediately after admission. What is the diagnosis?

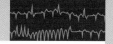

ANSWER 62

The ECG shows:
- Sinus rhythm, rate 140 bpm
- Normal conduction
- Normal axis
- Normal QRS complexes
- Slightly depressed ST segments in leads V_1–V_4
- Biphasic or inverted T waves in the inferior leads and all the chest leads.

Clinical interpretation

The ECG shows a marked sinus tachycardia, with no change in the cardiac axis and normal QRS complexes. The widespread ST segment/T wave changes are clearly very abnormal, but are not specific for any particular disease. However, the fact that leads V_1–V_3 are affected suggests a right ventricular problem.

The pulmonary angiogram shows a large central pulmonary embolus and occlusion of the arteries to the right lower lung.

What to do

This is a case where the ECG must be considered in the light of the patient's history and physical signs (if any). Clearly something has happened: the sudden onset of breathlessness without pain suggests a central pulmonary embolus – with pulmonary emboli that do not reach the pleural surface of the lung there may be little pain. In this patient, an echocardiogram and then a pulmonary angiogram demonstrated a large pulmonary embolus. Remember that sudden breathlessness with clear lung fields on a routine chest X-ray is always assumed to be due to a pulmonary embolus until proved otherwise. Anticoagulation is essential; thrombolysis should be considered.

SUMMARY

Sinus tachycardia with widespread ST segment/T wave changes, suggesting pulmonary embolism.

 See *ECG Made Easy*, 9th edition, Chapter 7

ECG 63

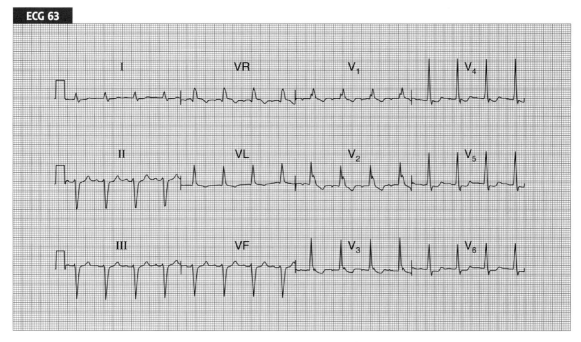

A 70-year-old man is sent to the clinic because of rather vague attacks of dizziness, which occur approximately once per week. Otherwise he is well, and there are no abnormalities on examination. Does this ECG help with his management?

ANSWER 63

The ECG shows:
- Sinus rhythm, rate 94 bpm
- PR interval at the upper limit of normal (200 ms)
- Left axis deviation
- QRS complex duration prolonged (160 ms)
- RSR^1 pattern in leads V_1–V_2; wide S wave in lead V_6
- Inverted T waves in leads VL, V_1–V_4.

Clinical interpretation

The left axis deviation is characteristic of left anterior hemiblock. There is also right bundle branch block (RBBB), so two of the main conducting pathways are blocked, resulting in 'bifascicular block'. The fact that the PR interval is at the upper limit of normal raises the possibility of delayed conduction in the remaining pathway; if the PR interval were definitely prolonged, this would indicate 'trifascicular block'.

What to do

Bifascicular block is not an indication for pacing if the patient is asymptomatic. The problem here is to decide if the attacks of dizziness are due to intermittent higher degree AV block causing bradyarrhythmias. Ideally an ECG would be recorded during an attack. Since they occur only every week or so, a longer period of ambulatory ECG recording will be required to capture an episode. A loop recorder (whether external or implanted) might be the best approach.

SUMMARY

Left anterior hemiblock and RBBB – bifascicular block.

 See *ECG Made Easy*, 9th edition, Chapter 3

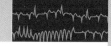

ECG 64

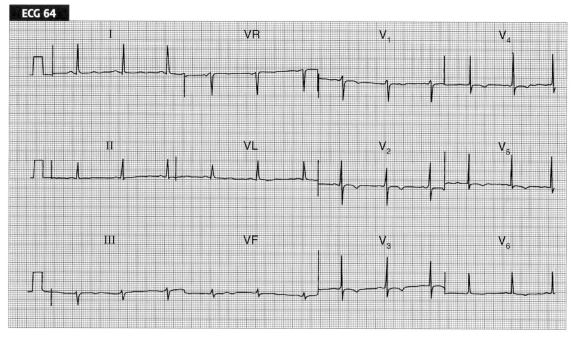

This ECG was recorded from a 25-year-old black professional footballer. What does it show, and what would you do?

ANSWER 64

The ECG shows:

- Sinus rhythm, rate 61 bpm
- Normal axis
- Normal QRS complexes
- Widespread T wave inversion, particularly in leads V_2–V_5.

Clinical interpretation

Repolarization (T wave) abnormalities are quite common in people of African origin, but alternative explanations for this ECG appearance would be a non-ST segment elevation myocardial infarction (unlikely in this clinical context), or a cardiomyopathy.

What to do

This man is a professional football player, so it is important to exclude hypertrophic cardiomyopathy, and this can be done by echocardiography. Because his career depended upon coronary disease being excluded, a coronary angiogram was performed and was entirely normal.

SUMMARY

Widespread T wave inversion, probably normal in a man of African origin.

 See *ECG Made Easy*, 9th edition, Chapter 6

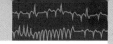

ECG 65

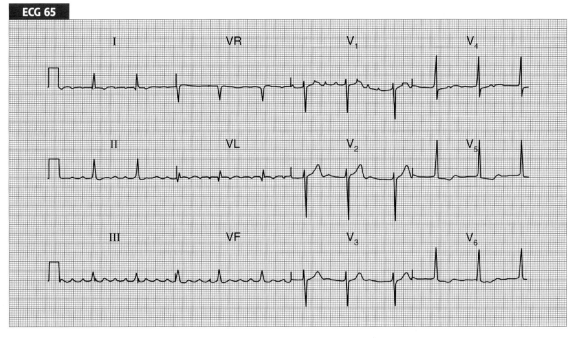

A 60-year-old woman is seen in the outpatient department, complaining of breathlessness. There are no abnormal physical findings. What does this ECG show, what might be the underlying problem and how would you treat her?

ANSWER 65

The ECG shows:
- Atrial flutter, best seen in lead III
- 4:1 block
- Normal axis
- Normal QRS complexes
- Sloping ST segment depression, best seen in leads V_5–V_6.

Clinical interpretation

This shows atrial flutter with what appears to be a stable 4:1 block. The ST segment depression is non-specific or could relate to digoxin use.

What to do

The stable 4:1 block has caused a regular heartbeat, so the arrhythmia was not suspected at the time of the clinical examination. There is nothing in this ECG to indicate the underlying disease, which could be ischaemic or rheumatic heart disease, or a cardiomyopathy: echocardiography is needed. The downward-sloping ST segments suggest digoxin treatment. Digoxin is not generally the first-line medication for rate control but can still be useful where blood pressure limits use of other drugs (such as beta-blockers) or as a second-line agent where rate control is not achieved with a single drug. If managed without cardioversion, her CHA2DS2-VASc score (or similar assessment) should be used to assess the need for anticoagulation. However given her symptoms, cardioversion (following a period of anticoagulation) and even ultimately ablation therapy, should be considered.

> **SUMMARY**
>
> Atrial flutter with 4:1 block.

 See *ECG Made Easy*, 9th edition, Chapter 4

ECG 66

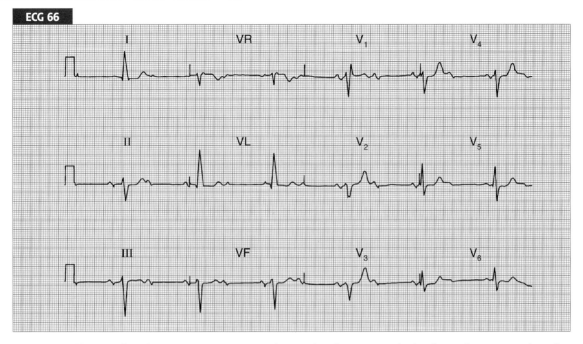

An 80-year-old man is found at routine examination to have a slow heart rate and a harsh systolic murmur. This is his ECG. What does it show, and what is the likely diagnosis? Is treatment necessary?

ANSWER 66

The ECG shows:
- Sinus rhythm, P wave rate 75 bpm
- Second degree (2:1) block
- Left axis deviation
- QRS complex duration 140 ms, with an RSR^1 pattern in lead V$_1$, indicating right bundle branch block (RBBB).

Clinical interpretation

This is second degree block and not complete (third degree) block. Left axis deviation (left anterior hemiblock) and RBBB constitute bifascicular block, but the 2:1 block shows that there is also significant disease in either the His bundle or the remaining posterior fascicle.

What to do

This patient needs a pacemaker. The combination of a heart murmur and heart block suggests aortic stenosis which is associated with AV node disease. The severity of this can be assessed with echocardiography.

> **SUMMARY**
>
> Second degree (2:1) block.

 See *ECG Made Easy*, 9th edition, Chapter 3

ECG 67

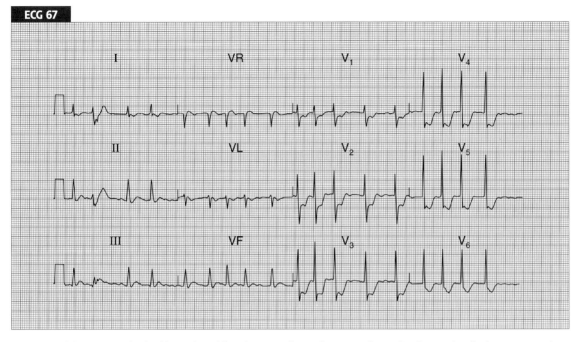

A 70-year-old woman, who had been breathless for several months, was admitted to hospital with chest pain, and this is her ECG. What does it show and what would you do?

ANSWER 67

The ECG shows:
- Atrial fibrillation, with one ventricular extrasystole
- Ventricular rate about 110 bpm
- Normal axis
- Normal QRS complexes
- Horizontal ST segment depression of 7 mm in lead V_2
- Downward-sloping ST segment depression in leads V_3–V_6
- Inverted T waves in leads I, VL, V_6; indeterminate T waves elsewhere.

Clinical interpretation

The anterior horizontal ST segment depression indicates severe ischaemia, which is presumably the cause of the chest pain. The ventricular rate is not too fast, and although the heart rate may be contributing to the ischaemia, it seems unlikely that it is the main problem. The most likely diagnosis is an acute coronary syndrome leading to a non ST elevation myocardial infarction (NSTEMI). This will be confirmed by measuring high sensitivity troponin.

What to do

The patient should be treated for an NSTEMI with dual antiplatelet therapy (aspirin and, in this instance, clopidogrel may be the best option as long-term anticoagulation for atrial fibrillation may be needed), anticoagulation (e.g. with a low molecular weight heparin or fondaparinux), a beta-blocker and nitrates (initially buccal or sublingual, then intravenous). If the pain does not settle, early angiography with a view to revascularization by a coronary artery bypass graft (CABG) or percutaneous coronary intervention (PCI) will have to be considered.

SUMMARY

Atrial fibrillation and anterior ischaemia.

 See *ECG Made Easy*, 9th edition, Chapter 7

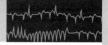

ECG 68

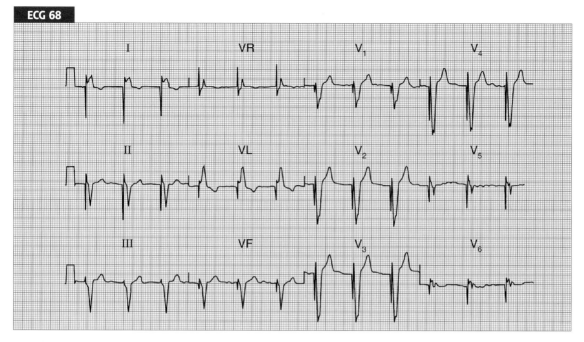

An elderly woman is admitted to hospital unconscious, evidently having had a stroke. No cardiac abnormalities are noted, but this is her ECG. What has been missed?

ANSWER 68

The ECG shows:

- No P waves; irregular baseline suggesting atrial fibrillation
- Regular QRS complexes; rate 73 bpm
- Left axis deviation
- Wide QRS complexes of an indeterminate pattern, with inverted T waves in some leads
- Each QRS complex is preceded by a deep and narrow spike.

Clinical interpretation

The narrow spike is due to a pacemaker, and someone has not noticed the permanent pacing battery, which is probably below the left clavicle. The pacing wire will be stimulating the right ventricle, giving rise to broad QRS complexes resembling a bundle branch block pattern. The underlying rhythm here is atrial fibrillation: the patient may have had atrial fibrillation with a slow ventricular response or complete AV block, or may have developed atrial fibrillation since pacing for another indication.

What to do

If this patient was not anticoagulated, the stroke may well have been due to an embolus arising in the left heart as a result of atrial fibrillation. If she was anticoagulated for her atrial fibrillation, an intracranial haemorrhage is possible. Either way she requires urgent brain imaging. Management for acute stroke may include thrombolysis or percutaneous intervention depending on local practice and in accordance with guidelines. Anticoagulation for her atrial fibrillation may be appropriate later depending on her response to initial treatment.

SUMMARY

Ventricular-paced rhythm and atrial fibrillation.

 See *ECG Made Easy*, 9th edition, Chapter 8

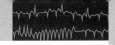

ECG 69

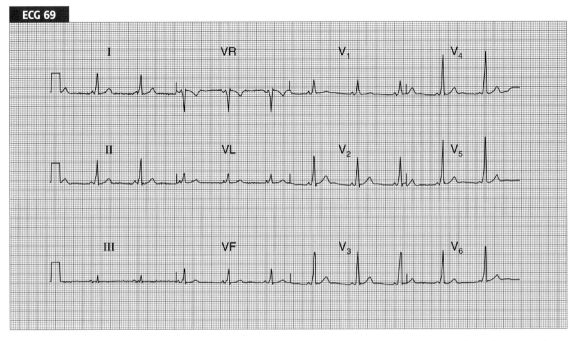

A 30-year-old woman, who had a baby 3 months previously, complains of breathlessness, and this is her ECG. What is the problem?

ANSWER 69

The ECG shows:

- Sinus rhythm, rate 64 bpm
- Short PR interval at 100 ms
- Normal axis
- Normal QRS complex duration
- Slurred upstroke to QRS complexes (delta wave)
- Dominant R wave in lead V_1
- Normal ST segments and T waves.

Clinical interpretation

This ECG shows the Wolff–Parkinson–White (WPW) syndrome type A, which is characterized by a dominant R wave in lead V_1. This is likely to be coincidental to her presentation.

What to do

The catch here is that the dominant R wave in lead V_1 may be mistakenly thought to be due to right ventricular hypertrophy. In a young woman who complains of breathlessness after a pregnancy, pulmonary embolism is obviously a possibility, and this might well cause ECG evidence of right ventricular hypertrophy – but in the presence of the WPW syndrome this would be very difficult to diagnose from the ECG. The only thing that might help the diagnosis in this scenario would be the appearance of right axis deviation, which is not usually present in WPW syndrome, but is not present here. The differential diagnosis remains broad and other causes of breathlessness, such as anaemia, should also be considered. Further investigation will be required both for her breathlessness and for her WPW which may require an electrophysiological assessment.

> **SUMMARY**
>
> The WPW syndrome type A.

 See *ECG Made Easy*, 9th edition, Chapter 4

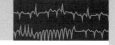

ECG 70

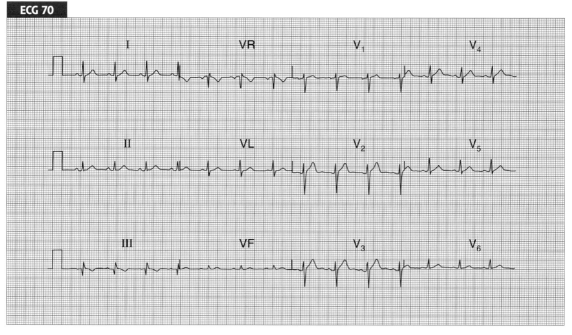

This ECG was recorded from a 60-year-old man with no symptoms, who wanted a private pilot's licence. Is the ECG normal? What would you tell the licensing authority?

ANSWER 70

The ECG shows:
- Sinus rhythm, rate 88 bpm
- Normal conduction
- Normal axis
- Q wave in lead III but not in lead VF
- Inverted T wave in lead III but not in lead VF
- U waves in leads V_2–V_3 (normal).

Clinical interpretation

A Q wave and/or an inverted T wave in lead III, but not in lead VF, is a normal variant. If lead III is recorded with the patient taking a deep breath in, the changes will often normalize as shown below.

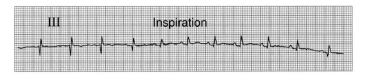

SUMMARY

Normal variant with Q waves and inverted T waves in lead III.

 See *ECG Made Easy*, 9th edition, Chapter 6

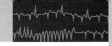

ECG 71

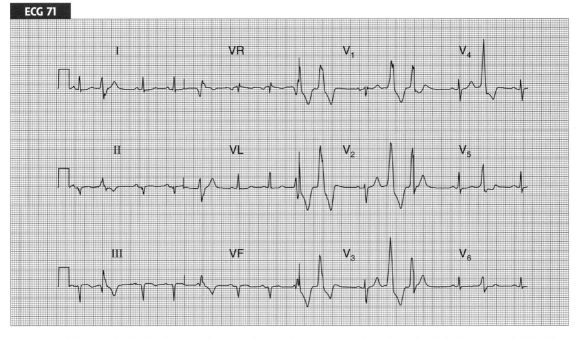

A 70-year-old man, who had had angina for several years, began to complain of attacks of dizziness. This is his ECG. What does it show and what would you do?

ANSWER 71

The ECG shows:
- Sinus rhythm, rate 88 bpm, with frequent multifocal ventricular extrasystoles
- Normal PR interval
- Normal axis
- Q waves in leads II, III, VF
- T waves flattened or inverted in the sinus beats in leads II, III, V_5–V_6.

Clinical interpretation

The ECG shows a probable old inferior myocardial infarction, so ischaemic heart disease accounts for his angina. Ventricular extrasystoles are in themselves usually not important, but in a patient complaining of attacks of dizziness, ventricular extrasystoles that are frequent and multifocal may be causing haemodynamic impairment.

What to do

It would be worth recording an ambulatory ECG to see if the patient is having runs of ventricular tachycardia, but the extrasystoles probably do need suppressing. A beta-blocker would be the first drug to try. If not previously assessed, his ischaemic heart disease and left ventricular function should be investigated and guideline-based therapy initiated. Cardiac stress MRI would cover both angles if locally available. Ultimately if angina is intrusive despite medical therapy and/or ischaemia on imaging is extensive, angiography with a view to revascularization may be appropriate.

> **SUMMARY**
>
> Old inferior myocardial infarction and frequent multifocal ventricular extrasystoles.

 See *ECG Made Easy*, 9th edition, Chapter 4

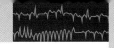

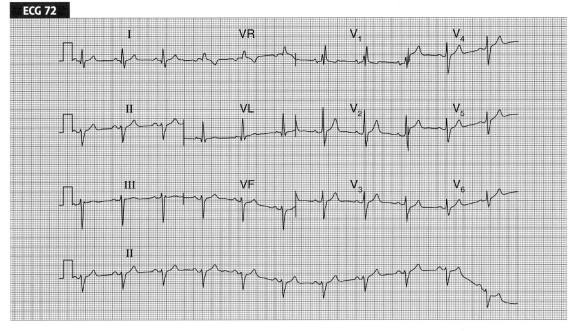

This ECG was recorded from a fit 60-year-old man at a routine medical examination. What does it show and what would you recommend?

ANSWER 72

The ECG shows:
- Sinus rhythm, rate 65 bpm
- Normal PR interval
- Left axis deviation – left anterior hemiblock
- QRS complex duration just over 120 ms, with an RSR^1 complex in lead V$_1$ – right bundle branch block (RBBB).

Clinical interpretation

The combination of left anterior hemiblock and RBBB is called bifascicular block. Atrioventricular conduction occurs via the posterior fascicle of the left bundle branch.

What to do

Progression to complete block can occur but is relatively rare. In the absence of symptoms, he does not require further investigation or a permanent pacemaker; however, any symptoms suggestive of a bradycardia should be investigated immediately.

SUMMARY

Left axis deviation and RBBB – bifascicular block.

 See *ECG Made Easy*, 9th edition, Chapter 3

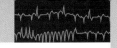

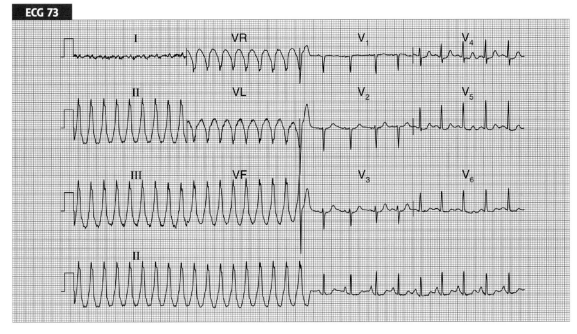

A 60-year-old man had complained of occasional episodes of palpitations for several years. Between attacks he was well, there were no physical abnormalities, and his ECG was normal. Eventually this ECG was recorded during one of his attacks. What is the arrhythmia and what would you do?

ANSWER 73

The lead II rhythm strip at the bottom of the record shows that the rhythm changes halfway through the recording, and this makes interpretation difficult. However, the ECG shows:

- Regular broad complex tachycardia, rate 160 bpm, followed by sinus rhythm, rate 120 bpm
- Normal axis during the tachycardia
- Broad QRS complexes, duration 160 ms
- QRS complexes normal during sinus rhythm
- During sinus rhythm there is ST segment depression in leads V_4–V_5.

Clinical interpretation

Without a full 12-lead record of the tachycardia it is difficult to be certain, but the complexes are very broad and have a totally different appearance from those in sinus rhythm, so this is almost certainly ventricular tachycardia. The ST segment depression in sinus rhythm is mild and not sufficient to make a confident diagnosis of ischaemia, but because the depression is horizontal, ischaemia seems likely.

What to do

Patients who have only occasional episodes of an arrhythmia, and who are otherwise well, are always difficult to manage. This patient should certainly have an echocardiogram to exclude a cardiomyopathy, and a perfusion scan and possibly a coronary angiogram to investigate the possibility of ischaemia. The arrhythmia seems to be exercise-induced and ambulatory monitoring would be worthwhile to see how frequently it occurs, and a very cautious exercise test might be justified to see how easily it is provoked. A specialist electrophysiological assessment with a view to ablation therapy should be considered before initiation of antiarrhythmic therapy. If the episodes were causing syncope, an implanted defibrillator could be considered.

> **SUMMARY**
>
> Paroxysmal ventricular tachycardia.

 See *ECG Made Easy*, 9th edition, Chapter 4

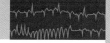

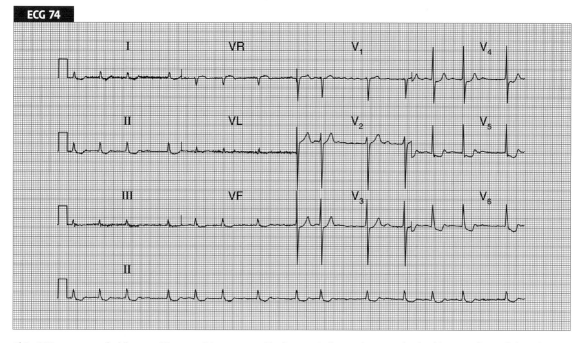

This ECG was recorded from a 60-year-old woman with rheumatic heart disease. She had been in heart failure, but this had been treated and she was no longer breathless. What does the ECG show, and what question might you ask her?

ANSWER 74

The ECG shows:
- Atrial fibrillation with a ventricular rate of about 80 bpm
- Normal axis
- Normal QRS complexes
- Downward-sloping ST segments, best seen in leads V_5–V_6
- Prominent U waves in leads V_2–V_3.

Clinical interpretation

The downward-sloping ST segments (the 'reverse tick') indicate that digoxin has been given (although this is no longer first-line treatment for rate control of atrial fibrillation). The ventricular rate seems well controlled. The prominent U waves in leads V_2–V_3 are probably normal: U waves due to hypokalaemia are associated with flattened T waves.

What to do

Ask the patient about her appetite: the earliest symptom of digoxin toxicity is appetite loss, followed by nausea and vomiting. If the patient is being treated with diuretics, check the serum potassium level – a low potassium level potentiates the effects of digoxin. If in doubt, the serum digoxin level is easily measured. It is important to appreciate that the presence of typical digoxin-related ECG changes is not diagnostic of digoxin toxicity. This is a clinical and biochemical diagnosis.

> **SUMMARY**
>
> Atrial fibrillation with digoxin effect.

 See *ECG Made Easy*, 9th edition, Chapter 4

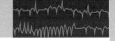

ECG 75

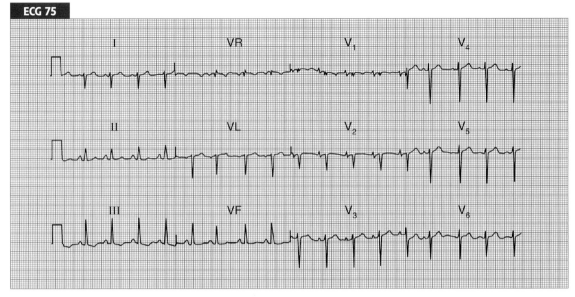

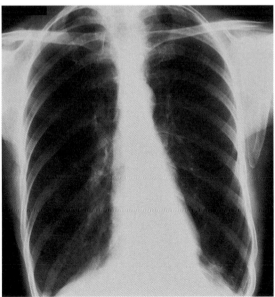

This ECG and chest X-ray were recorded from a 70-year-old man who complained of breathlessness. What abnormalities do they show and what is the most likely diagnosis? (X-ray reproduced with permission from Corne J & Pointon K (eds), *100 Chest X-Ray Problems*, Elsevier, 2007.)

ANSWER 75

The ECG shows:
- Sinus rhythm, rate 102 bpm
- Peaked P waves, best seen in leads V_1–V_2
- Right axis deviation (deep S waves in lead I)
- RSR[1] pattern with normal QRS complex duration in lead V_1 (partial right bundle branch block [RBBB])
- Deep S waves in lead V_6, with no left ventricular pattern.

The chest X-ray shows a long and thin mediastinum, with no increase in heart size but possible prominence of the pulmonary arteries. The lung fields appear essentially black, which is a feature of emphysema. This is the picture of chronic obstructive pulmonary disease (COPD).

Clinical interpretation

Peaked P waves suggest right atrial hypertrophy. The partial RBBB pattern is not significant. Right axis deviation may be seen in tall, thin people with normal hearts, but with the deep S waves in lead V_6 it suggests right ventricular hypertrophy. The lack of development of a left ventricular pattern in the V leads (i.e. deep S waves persisting into lead V_6) results from the right ventricle occupying most of the precordium. This is sometimes called 'clockwise rotation' (looking at the heart from below) and is characteristic of chronic lung disease.

What to do

Lung function tests may be more helpful than echocardiography but remember both COPD and heart disease are common and not infrequently occur in the same patient.

SUMMARY

Right atrial hypertrophy and chronic obstructive pulmonary disease.

 See *ECG Made Easy*, 9th edition, Chapter 7

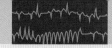

Part 2
More Challenging ECGs

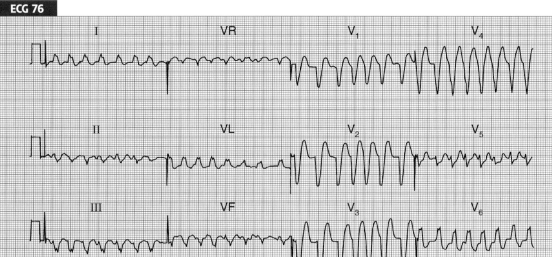

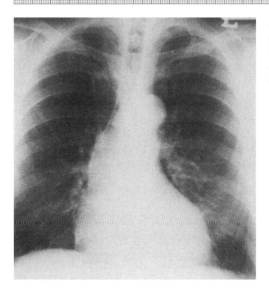

An 80-year-old man was admitted to hospital because of a sudden onset of palpitations associated with breathlessness. He had congestive cardiac failure and a heart murmur suggestive of aortic regurgitation. What do this ECG and the chest X-ray show, and how would you treat him?

ANSWER 76

The ECG shows:

- Broad complex tachycardia
- Irregular rhythm, rate 130–200 bpm
- No clear P waves but irregular baseline, best seen in lead VL
- QRS complex duration 160 ms, with 'M' pattern in lead V_6, indicating left bundle branch block (LBBB).

The chest X-ray shows left ventricular enlargement with dilatation of the ascending aorta. There is calcification in the aortic wall (arrowed). In this rare case, these changes suggest aortic regurgitation due to old syphilitic aortitis.

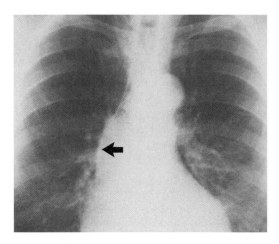

Clinical interpretation

The marked irregularity of rhythm, coupled with the irregular baseline glimpsed in one beat in lead VL, shows that this is atrial fibrillation with LBBB.

What to do

Aortic valve disease is commonly associated with LBBB as the aortic valve is anatomically close to the AV node. An echocardiogram is needed, to ensure that there is no significant aortic stenosis – in which case vasodilators (including ACE inhibitors) must be used with caution. The heart failure can be treated with diuretics. Cautious betablockade will control the ventricular rate. Once stabilized, consideration should be given to the risk-benefit of valve surgery or intervention.

SUMMARY

Atrial fibrillation with LBBB; aortic regurgitation due to syphilitic aortitis.

See *ECG Made Practical*, 7th edition, Chapter 4

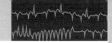

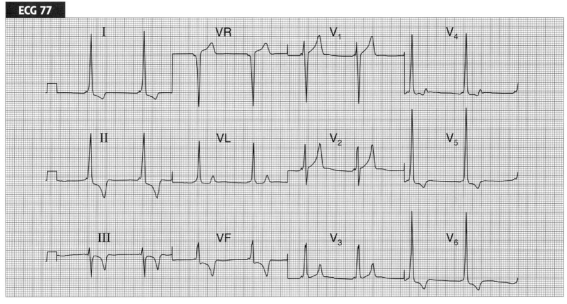

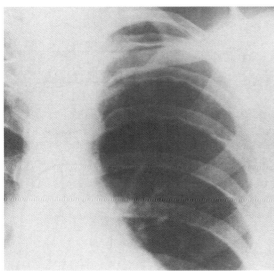

This ECG was recorded from a 35-year-old man who had no symptoms, but who had been found at a routine examination to have a blood pressure of 180/105. An enlarged part of the chest X-ray is also shown. What do the ECG and X-ray show and what action would you suggest?

ANSWER 77

The ECG (*note*: leads at half sensitivity) shows:
- Sinus rhythm, rate 50 bpm
- Very short PR interval
- Normal axis
- Slurred upstroke to QRS complexes – delta wave
- QRS complex duration prolonged (200 ms)
- Very tall QRS complexes in the lateral leads
- Inverted T waves in leads I–III, VF, V_5–V_6.

The chest X-ray shows rib notching (arrowed), due to collaterals that have developed because of a coarctation of the aorta.

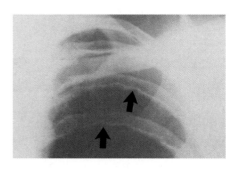

Clinical interpretation

The ECG shows an example of the Wolff–Parkinson–White (WPW) syndrome type B. In a patient with high blood pressure the tall QRS complexes and inverted T waves in the lateral leads would raise the possibility of left ventricular hypertrophy. However, the changes here are too gross for that, and they are compatible with this pre-excitation syndrome. The rib notching shows that the high blood pressure is due to coarctation of the aorta, which is completely unrelated to the WPW syndrome.

What to do

If the patient has no symptoms to suggest a paroxysmal tachycardia, no further action is necessary – many patients with an ECG consistent with a pre-excitation syndrome never have an episode of tachycardia. The chance finding of an unrelated coarctation of the aorta is more important, and surgical correction of this must be considered.

SUMMARY

The WPW syndrome type B, and an unrelated coarctation of the aorta.

See *ECG Made Practical*, 7th edition, Chapter 2

ECG 78

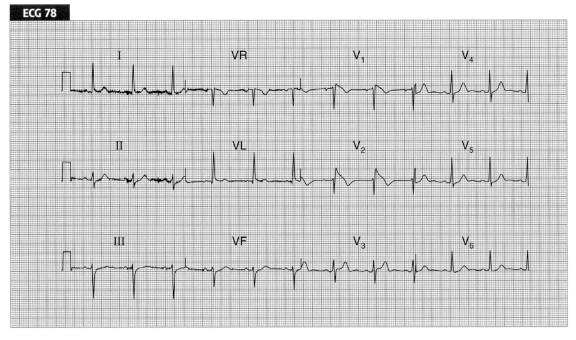

This ECG was recorded from a 40-year-old man who was admitted to hospital after collapsing in a supermarket. By the time he was seen he was well, and there were no abnormal physical signs. Would you pass this ECG as normal?

ANSWER 78

The ECG shows:
- Sinus rhythm, rate 70 bpm
- Normal PR interval and QRS complex duration
- Normal axis
- QRS complexes in leads V_1–V_2 show an RSR^1 pattern
- ST segments elevated, and downward-sloping, in leads V_1–V_2.

Clinical interpretation

This is not a normal ECG. The appearances in leads V_1–V_2 are characteristic of the Brugada syndrome.

What to do

The Brugada syndrome involves a genetic abnormality that alters sodium transport in the myocardium, and predisposes to ventricular tachycardia and fibrillation. This patient's collapse may well have been due to an arrhythmia. The syndrome can be familial and both genetic testing and family screening are indicated. The ECG changes are not constant, and on the day after admission this patient's ECG was perfectly normal. The ECG changes can be induced, and ventricular tachycardia caused, by fever, alcohol and a number of drugs (see https://www.brugadadrugs.org/). Given the history of syncope, this patient requires an implanted defibrillator.

SUMMARY

The Brugada syndrome.

 See *ECG Made Practical*, 7th edition, Chapter 2

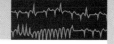

ECG 79

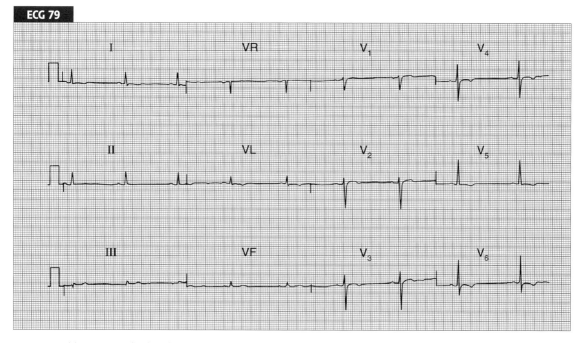

A 30-year-old woman, who had been treated for depression for several years, was admitted to hospital as an emergency following deliberate self-harm involving a small number of aspirin tablets. There were no abnormalities on examination, but this was her ECG. Does it worry you?

ANSWER 79

The ECG shows:
- Sinus rhythm, rate 50 bpm
- Normal axis
- Normal QRS complexes
- T wave inversion in leads I, VL, V_4–V_6.

Clinical interpretation

Anterolateral T wave inversion is most commonly due to ischaemia, but this seems unlikely in a young woman with no evidence of heart disease. A cardiomyopathy would be another possibility, but repolarization (T wave) abnormalities can be caused by lithium therapy.

What to do

As always when a diagnosis is not clear, find out what drugs the patient is taking. This patient was taking lithium, and exercise testing and echocardiography showed no evidence of heart disease.

SUMMARY

Anterolateral T wave inversion due to lithium therapy.

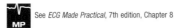 See *ECG Made Practical*, 7th edition, Chapter 8

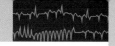

ECG 80

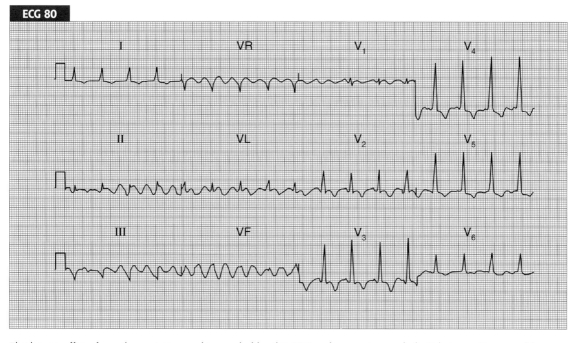

The house officer from the geriatric ward is puzzled by this ECG and requests your help. What questions would you ask him?

ECG 80

ANSWER 80

The ECG shows:
- Sinus rhythm, rate 100 bpm
- Slow rhythmic waves, the baseline in some ways resembling atrial flutter, but slower and coarser
- Short PR intervals
- Slurred upstroke of the QRS complexes, particularly in lead I
- T wave inversion in the anterior leads.

Clinical interpretation

The slow rhythmic variation is due to muscle tremor, and is not cardiac in origin. The short PR intervals, slurred upstroke of the QRS complexes and inverted T waves are due to the Wolff–Parkinson–White (WPW) syndrome – the dominant R waves in the chest leads indicating type A.

What to do

Ask if the patient has Parkinson's disease: a Parkinsonian tremor would explain the baseline variation. Does the patient give a history of palpitations or syncope? This would be the only significant problem that the WPW syndrome might cause in an elderly patient.

SUMMARY

Muscle artefact, possibly Parkinson's disease; the WPW syndrome type A.

 See *ECG Made Practical*, 7th edition, Chapters 2 and 4

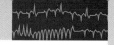

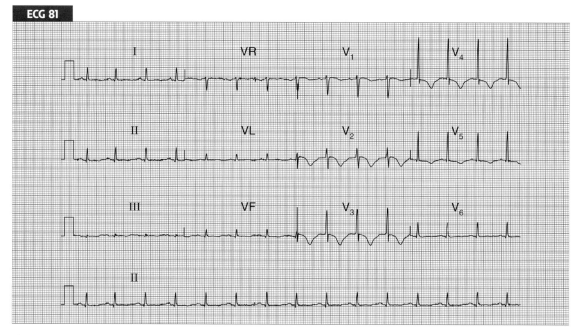

This ECG was recorded from a 15-year-old boy who collapsed while playing football. His brother had died suddenly. What does the ECG show and what clinical possibilities should be considered?

ANSWER 81

The ECG shows:
- Sinus rhythm, rate 91 bpm
- Normal PR interval
- Normal axis
- Normal QRS complexes
- Prolonged QT interval (QT=492 ms; QT_c=598 ms)
- Inverted T waves in leads V_2–V_5.

Clinical interpretation

This is clearly a very abnormal ECG, with a markedly prolonged QT interval and abnormal T waves.

What to do

The family history suggests that this may well be an example of one of the congenital forms of prolonged QT interval. These are characterized by episodes of loss of consciousness in children, often at times of increased sympathetic nervous system activity, and beta-blockers are the immediate form of treatment. The insertion of a permanent defibrillator should be considered. Prolonged QT interval syndrome is also associated with antiarrhythmic drugs (including amiodarone and sotalol) and with other drugs such as the tricyclic antidepressants and erythromycin. Electrolyte abnormalities (low potassium, magnesium or calcium levels) also prolong the QT interval.

SUMMARY

Marked prolongation of the QT interval – long QT syndrome.

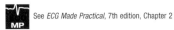 See *ECG Made Practical*, 7th edition, Chapter 2

ECG 82

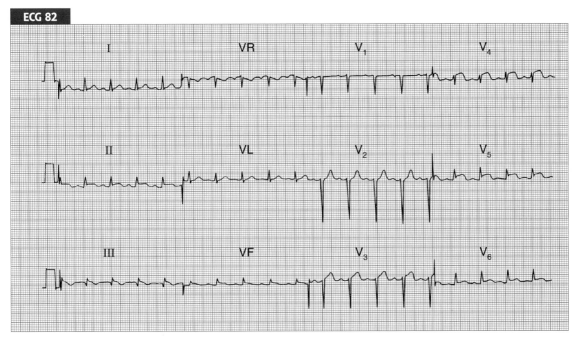

This ECG was recorded in the A&E department from a 25-year-old man with severe chest pain. No physical abnormalities had been detected, but having seen the ECG, what would you look for and what would you do?

ANSWER 82

The ECG shows:
- Sinus rhythm, rate 105 bpm
- Normal axis
- Normal QRS complexes
- Raised ST segments in leads I–III, VF, V_4–V_6.

Clinical interpretation

The raised ST segments could indicate an acute infarction, but since the change is so widespread, is not in a particular coronary territory and shows no reciprocal ST-depresssion, pericarditis seems much more probable.

What to do

In a 25-year-old, pericarditis is a much more likely diagnosis than infarction. When lying the patient flat, a pericardial rub may become much easier to hear but is not always present. Echocardiography will confirm no myocardial regional wall motion abnormality and may show a pericardial effusion if one is present. Management is with non-steroidal anti-inflammatory drugs and colchicine.

> **SUMMARY**
>
> Widespread ST segment elevation, suggesting pericarditis.

 See *ECG Made Practical*, 7th edition, Chapter 6

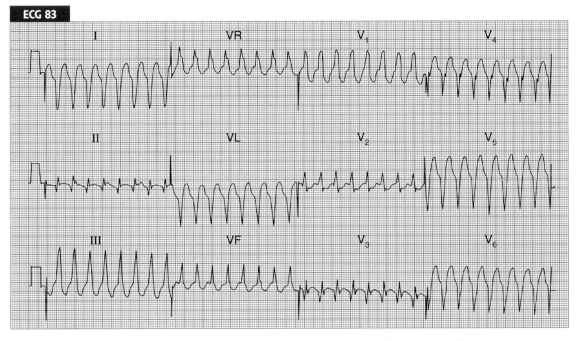

A 45-year-old man was admitted to hospital with a history of 2 h of ischaemic chest pain. His blood pressure was 150/80, and there were no signs of heart failure. What does his ECG show, and how would you treat him?

ANSWER 83

The ECG shows:
- Broad complex tachycardia, rate 180 bpm
- No P waves
- Right axis deviation
- QRS complex duration about 140 ms
- Right bundle branch block (RBBB) pattern, with the R peak taller than the R^1 peak in lead V_1 – best seen in the fifth complex
- Non-concordant QRS complexes, with a negative pattern in lead V_6 (i.e. complexes are upwards in lead V_1 but downwards in lead V_6).

Clinical interpretation

This is either ventricular tachycardia or supraventricular tachycardia with RBBB. In favour of the former are the relatively wide QRS complexes and the fact that the R peak is greater than the R^1 peak in lead V_1 (i.e. this is not the typical RBBB pattern). Against ventricular tachycardia are the right axis deviation and the different directions of the QRS complexes in the chest leads.

What to do

To some extent agonizing about the underlying arrhythmia here is unnecessary. The most sensible strategy is to call an anaesthetist and arrange urgent DC cardioversion. In the interim, intravenous adenosine could be cautiously tried providing the blood pressure remains adequate and there is no history of asthma.

This patient underwent cardioversion, and the ECG then showed an anterior infarction. The rhythm was probably ventricular tachycardia.

SUMMARY

Broad complex tachycardia – probably ventricular tachycardia.

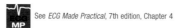 See *ECG Made Practical*, 7th edition, Chapter 4

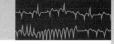

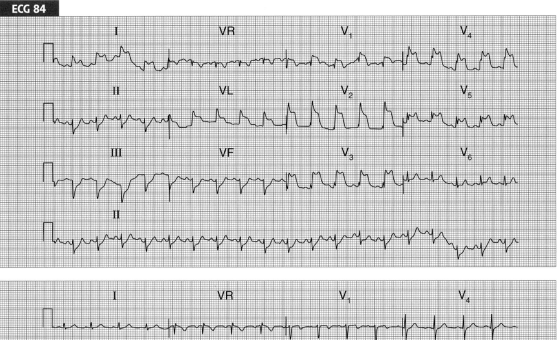

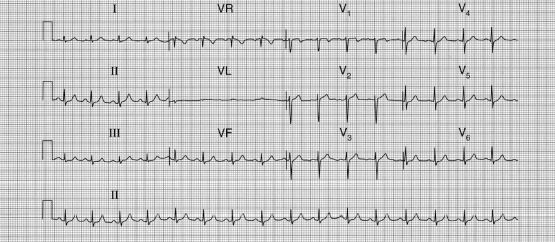

The upper ECG was recorded by paramedics from a 50-year-old woman who had had episodes of chest pain for several years, and who called an ambulance because of a severe attack. By the time she reached the A&E department, when the lower ECG was recorded, her pain had gone. What had happened?

171

ANSWER 84

The upper ECG shows:
- Sinus rhythm, average rate 111 bpm
- Left axis deviation
- QRS complexes probably normal, but partly obscured by the ST segments
- Raised ST segments in leads I, VL, V$_1$–V$_5$
- T waves probably normal.

The lower ECG shows:
- Sinus rhythm, rate 97 bpm
- Normal axis
- Normal QRS complexes, ST segments and T waves.

Clinical interpretation

The first ECG seems to indicate an acute anterolateral myocardial infarction. An alternative explanation, given the widespread changes, would be pericarditis. The second ECG is normal. Because the ECG reverted to normal when the pain cleared, it seems likely that the changes in the initial ECG represent ischaemia. In this case coronary angiography showed no obstructive coronary disease. This was a case of Prinzmetal's variant angina.

What to do

Prinzmetal's variant angina was first described in 1959. It occurs at rest, and the characteristic raised ST segments seen in the ECG are not reproduced by exertion. It has been shown by angiography during pain to be due to spasm of one or more coronary arteries. Relatively few patients with this type of angina have totally normal arteries, and spasm may occur at the site of atheromatous plaques. Vasodilator therapies may be helpful, but the condition can be difficult to treat.

SUMMARY

Prinzmetal's variant angina.

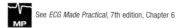 See *ECG Made Practical*, 7th edition, Chapter 6

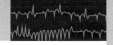
ECG 85

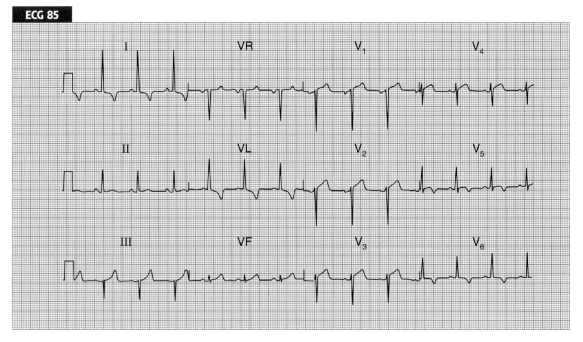

A 50-year-old man complains of typical angina. His blood pressure is 150/90, and he has an aortic ejection systolic murmur. This is his ECG. What is the probable cause of his angina, and what would you do?

ANSWER 85

The ECG shows:

- Sinus rhythm, rate 77 bpm
- Normal axis
- Normal QRS complexes
- Raised ST segments following S waves in leads V_4–V_5
- Inverted T waves in leads I, VL, V_5–V_6.

Clinical interpretation

The raised ST segments in leads V_4–V_5 are due to 'high take-off' and are not important. The lateral T wave inversion could indicate left ventricular hypertrophy or ischaemia, and this patient could have aortic stenosis or coronary disease. In the absence of tall R waves, lateral ischaemia seems more likely than left ventricular hypertrophy, but it is often difficult to distinguish between these on the ECG.

What to do

Echocardiography will show whether the patient has significant aortic valve disease. Once this has been excluded, further investigations for coronary artery disease are indicated. Remember also that anaemia can cause systolic murmurs and angina, although probably not this degree of T wave inversion. This patient had coronary disease.

SUMMARY

Probable lateral ischaemia, but possible left ventricular hypertrophy.

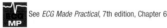 See *ECG Made Practical*, 7th edition, Chapter 6

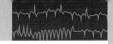

ECG 86

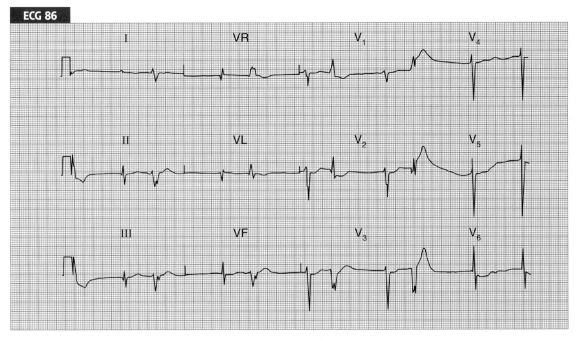

A 60-year-old woman, with long-standing heart failure of uncertain cause, complains of anorexia, weight loss, and general weakness and lethargy. Does this ECG help with her diagnosis and management?

ANSWER 86

The ECG shows:
- Atrial fibrillation
- Coupled ventricular extrasystoles
- Q waves in lead VL (in the supraventricular beats)
- ST segment depression in lead V_6
- Flattened T waves and prominent U waves (best seen in lead V_4).

Clinical interpretation

Heart failure per se can cause anorexia, weakness and weight loss. The patient will be taking diuretics so assessment of electrolytes is required to exclude hypokalaemia. If the patient is taking digoxin, toxicity should be considered. The ECG findings in lead V_6 are consistent with a digoxin effect, and coupled ventricular extrasystoles could be features of digoxin toxicity. The flat T waves and prominent U waves may suggest hypokalaemia.

What to do

Check the electrolytes, and give oral potassium supplements if required. Guideline-based treatment for heart failure should be initiated. Betablockade may provide adequate rate control without the need for digoxin. A mineralocorticoid receptor antagonist could be considered both as treatment for heart failure and as a potassium-sparing diuretic.

SUMMARY

Atrial fibrillation with ventricular extrasystoles; probable digoxin toxicity and hypokalaemia.

 See *ECG Made Practical*, 7th edition, Chapter 8

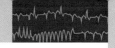
ECG 87

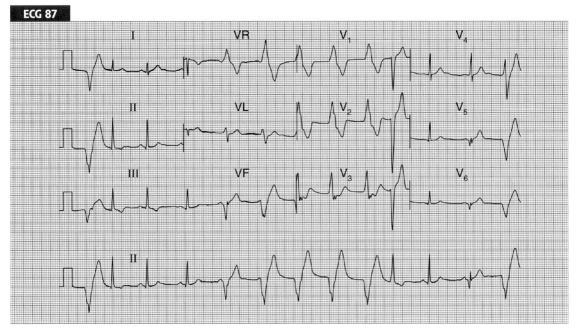

This ECG was recorded as part of the health screening of an asymptomatic 40-year-old man. How would you proceed?

ANSWER 87

The lead II rhythm strip at the bottom of the record shows that the rhythm changed during the recording, so it is necessary to try to identify the normal complexes (if any) in each lead. There are normal beats in the second and third complexes in leads I, II and III; in the first complex in leads VR, VL and VF; in the last complex in leads V_1–V_3; and in the first complex in leads V_4–V_6. The ECG shows:

- Sinus rhythm at about 77 bpm, with ventricular extrasystoles at the beginning and end of the record, and a six-beat run of a broad complex rhythm in the middle of the record
- The first complex of the run of broad complexes differs from the others, and is probably a fusion beat (a combination of a sinus beat and the ectopic rhythm)
- Normal axis when in sinus rhythm
- Normal QRS complexes in sinus rhythm
- Inverted T waves in lead III, but not VF.

Clinical interpretation

The run of broad complexes represents accelerated idioventricular rhythm. This is quite common following a myocardial infarction, but in a healthy subject it is probably of no significance. The T wave inversion in lead III is not important because the T wave is upright in lead VF.

What to do

Ambulatory ECG monitoring over 24 hours and confirmation of a structurally normal heart by echocardiography or cardiac MRI will provide reassurance. If the individual has no symptoms and the physical examination is otherwise normal, no further action is needed. Accelerated idioventricular rhythm should not be treated.

SUMMARY

Sinus rhythm and accelerated idioventricular rhythm.

 See *ECG Made Practical*, 7th edition, Chapter 1

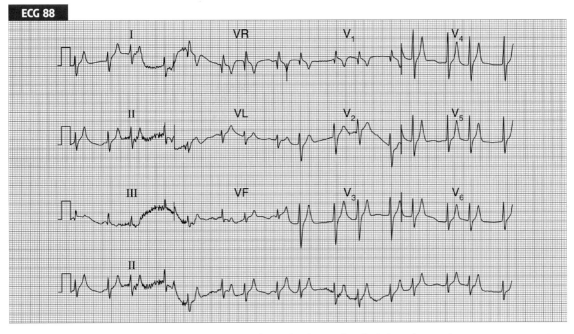

This ECG was recorded from a 30-year-old woman admitted to hospital with diabetic ketoacidosis. Any comments?

ANSWER 88

This is not a technically good record, and exhibits considerable artefacts. However, the ECG shows:

- The rhythm is probably sinus, with coupled junctional extrasystoles
- P waves difficult to identify, but there are probably flattened P waves before the first of each pair of QRS complexes, best seen in lead VR
- Probably normal PR interval
- Normal axis
- Narrow QRS complexes, so this is a supraventricular rhythm
- QRS complexes apparently in pairs, which are identical
- QRS complex duration at the upper limit of normal (120 ms)
- ST segment not easy to identify
- T waves sharply peaked in all leads.

Clinical interpretation

These changes are characteristic of hyperkalaemia, which of course is likely to be secondary to diabetic ketoacidosis.

What to do

This ECG should alert you to check the serum potassium level immediately: in this patient, it was found to be 7.1 mmol/l. This degree of hyperkalaemia with ECG changes requires emergency treatment with calcium gluconate or calcium carbonate as well as treatment of the underlying dehydration and hyperglycaemia.

SUMMARY

Hyperkalaemia.

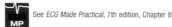 See *ECG Made Practical*, 7th edition, Chapter 8

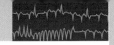
ECG 89

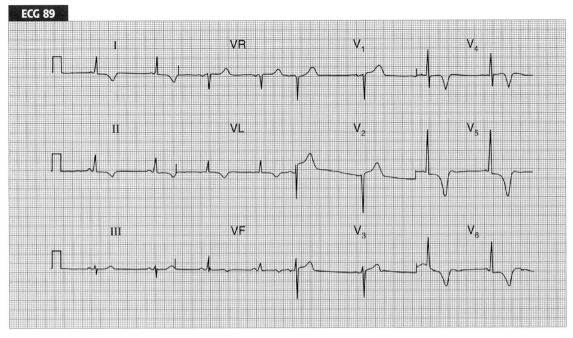

A 35-year-old white man is seen in the outpatient department complaining of chest pain on exertion, sometimes with exertion-induced dizziness, and this is his ECG. What is the likely diagnosis? What physical signs would you look for?

ANSWER 89

The ECG shows:
- Sinus rhythm
- Normal axis
- Normal QRS complexes
- Marked T wave inversion in leads I, II, VL, V_4–V_6.

Clinical interpretation

Anterolateral T wave inversion as gross as this may be due to a non-ST segment elevation myocardial infarction. However, on this trace the changes are due to left ventricular hypertrophy secondary to a hypertrophic cardiomyopathy. Myocardial infarction is uncommon in people of this age.

What to do

Physical signs of hypertrophic cardiomyopathy include a 'jerky pulse'; an aortic flow murmur which is characteristically louder after the pause that follows an extrasystole; and mitral regurgitation. Hypertrophic cardiomyopathy is best diagnosed by echocardiography or cardiac MRI, which will show asymmetric septal hypertrophy, systolic anterior movement of the mitral valve apparatus and sometimes associated left ventricular outflow tract obstruction and/or mitral regurgitation. This patient's echocardiogram showed all these features, confirming the diagnosis of hypertrophic cardiomyopathy.

> **SUMMARY**
>
> Gross T wave inversion in the anterolateral leads, suggesting hypertrophic cardiomyopathy.

 See *ECG Made Practical*, 7th edition, Chapters 2 and 6

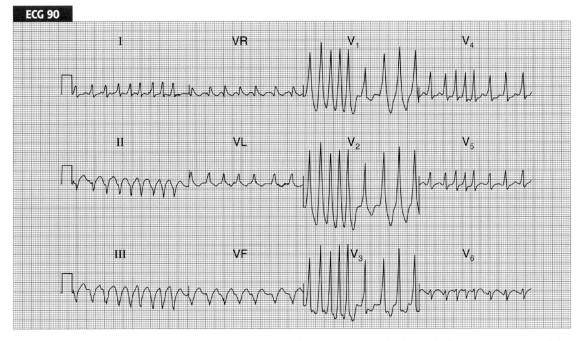

A 25-year-old woman, who had had episodes of what sound like a paroxysmal tachycardia for 10 years, produced this ECG when seen during an attack. What is the rhythm, and what is the underlying problem?

ANSWER 90

The ECG shows:
- Irregular tachycardia at about 200 bpm
- No consistent P waves visible
- Left axis deviation
- QRS complex duration varies between about 120 and 160 ms
- QRS complexes show a dominant R wave in lead V_1 and a prominent S wave in lead V_6
- After the longer pauses, the upstroke of the QRS complexes appears slurred.

Clinical interpretation

The marked irregularity of this rhythm must be explained by atrial fibrillation. The broad QRS complexes might be due to right bundle branch block, but the dominant R wave in lead V_1, together with the slurred upstroke of the QRS complex in at least some leads, indicate the Wolff–Parkinson–White (WPW) syndrome type A.

What to do

A combination of the WPW syndrome and atrial fibrillation is very dangerous, because it can degenerate into ventricular fibrillation. The arrhythmia needs treating as an emergency with DC cardioversion under sedation of anaesthesia, whatever the clinical state of the patient. It is important not to use drugs that may block the atrioventricular node (such as adenosine, verapamil or beta-blockers) as these increase conduction through the accessory pathway and increase the risk of ventricular fibrillation. Following cardioversion, flecainide can be used as an antiarrhythmic pending an electrophysiological study to identify and ablate the accessory pathway.

> **SUMMARY**
>
> Atrial fibrillation and the WPW syndrome type A.

 See *ECG Made Practical*, 7th edition, Chapter 4

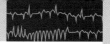

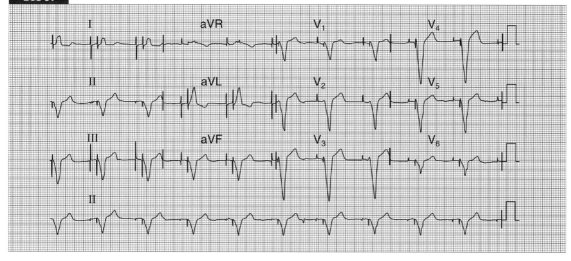

An elderly man was admitted unconscious after a stroke, and this was his ECG. Does it help with diagnosis and management?

ANSWER 91

The ECG shows:
- A regular broad complex rhythm at 60 bpm
- There is a sharp "pacing" spike immediately before each QRS
- P waves are not easy to see except perhaps in V_2, but there are pacing spikes where P waves would be expected.

Clinical interpretation

This ECG shows dual chamber (i.e., right atrial and right ventricular) pacing.

What to do

There is nothing on this ECG to suggest pacemaker malfunction and the underlying rhythm is probably sinus. The pacemaker is probably not related to the stroke.

> **SUMMARY**
>
> Dual chamber pacemaker.

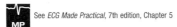 See *ECG Made Practical*, 7th edition, Chapter 5

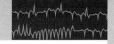

ECG 92

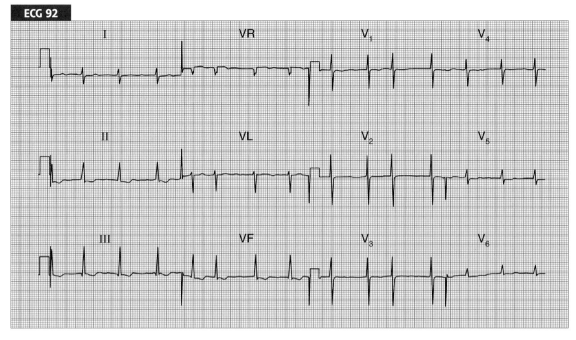

This ECG was recorded from a 65-year-old woman who had had a mitral valve replacement to treat rheumatic valve disease, and who was admitted to hospital with generalized lethargy, nausea and vomiting. What does the ECG show, and what would you do? Unfortunately, the chemical pathology laboratory burned down last night.

ANSWER 92

The ECG (*note*: chest leads at half sensitivity) shows:

- Atrial fibrillation
- Right axis deviation
- Normal QRS complexes, except for a tall R wave in lead V_1
- Downward-sloping ST segments, best seen in leads II, III, VF
- Generally flattened T waves
- U waves, best seen in leads V_4–V_5.

Clinical interpretation

The atrial fibrillation, and the right axis deviation and tall R waves in lead V_1 (indicating right ventricular hypertrophy) probably pre-date the valve replacement. The flat T waves with obvious U waves suggest hypokalaemia. The downward-sloping ST segments suggest digoxin effect.

What to do

The clinical picture fits hypokalaemia and digoxin toxicity. Since the electrolyte and digoxin levels cannot be measured, stop the digoxin and any potassium-losing diuretics. Once the serum potassium has been determined, give the patient potassium orally. Monitoring the T and U waves is a crude but effective way of judging the serum potassium level.

SUMMARY

Atrial fibrillation, hypokalaemia and digoxin effect.

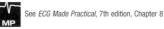 See *ECG Made Practical*, 7th edition, Chapter 8

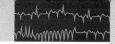

ECG 93

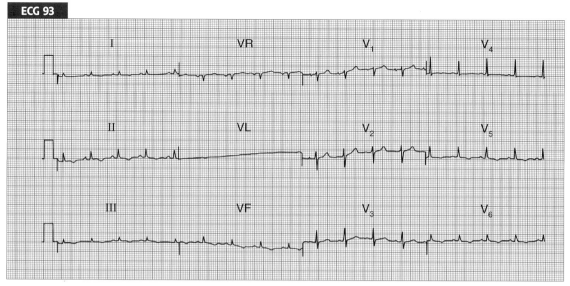

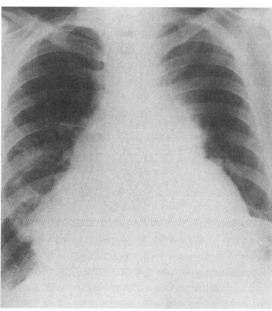

A 70-year-old man with lung cancer is admitted to hospital with abdominal pain and ankle swelling. He has a raised jugular venous pressure, a tender and distended liver, and marked peripheral oedema. Does this ECG help with the diagnosis and what might you need to do? What does the chest X-ray show?

ANSWER 93

The ECG shows:
- Sinus rhythm, rate 97 bpm
- Normal axis
- QRS complexes of normal width, but generally small
- T wave inversion in leads I, II, III, VF, V_5–V_6
- Loss of signal in lead VL – artefact.

The chest X-ray shows an enlarged cardiac shadow with a triangular shape, suggesting a pericardial effusion.

Clinical interpretation

Small QRS complexes are seen with a pericardial effusion, and sometimes in patients with chronic lung disease. The widespread T wave changes would be consistent with pericardial disease. There is nothing in this record to suggest pulmonary disease.

What to do

The physical findings, the ECG and the chest X-ray would fit with a pericardial effusion, potentially associated with malignancy. You should look carefully at the jugular venous pressure to see if it rises with inspiration, indicating pericardial tamponade. Echocardiography is essential, and if this confirms tamponade, a pericardial drain should be inserted as an emergency. The patient had a malignant pericardial effusion.

> **SUMMARY**
>
> Small QRS complexes and widespread T wave changes consistent with a pericardial effusion.

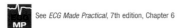 See *ECG Made Practical*, 7th edition, Chapter 6

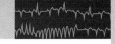

ECG 94

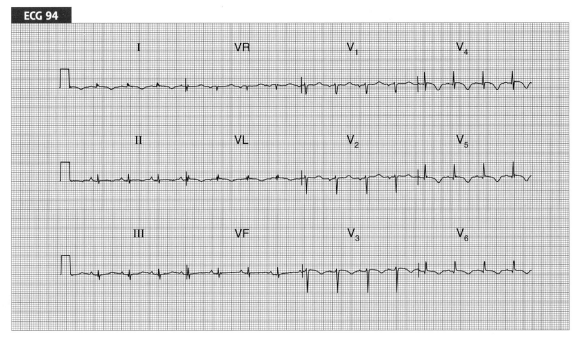

This ECG was recorded as part of the routine investigation of a 40-year-old man who was admitted to hospital following a first seizure. He was unconscious and had a stiff neck and bilateral extensor plantar responses. His heart was clinically normal. What do you think has happened?

ANSWER 94

This ECG shows:

- Sinus rhythm, rate 90 bpm
- Normal PR interval and QRS complex duration
- Normal axis
- Small Q waves in the lateral leads, probably septal
- Normal QRS complexes
- T wave inversion in leads I, VL, V_4–V_6
- Prolonged QT interval (QT_c=529 ms).

Clinical interpretation

The appearances here are suggestive of an anterolateral non-ST segment elevation myocardial infarction, but this does not correspond with the clinical picture and would not explain the long QT interval.

What to do

It is possible that this patient had a myocardial infarction which caused a cerebrovascular accident because of an arrhythmia or a cerebral embolus, and that the cerebrovascular accident caused the seizure. The unconsciousness and the bilateral extensor plantar responses could simply be post-ictal. However, such a sequence would not explain the stiff neck, which would seem to point to either a subarachnoid haemorrhage or meningitis. Changes like those in this ECG are common in subarachnoid haemorrhage. Measurements of the blood troponin level are unlikely to help to differentiate between a primarily cardiac and a primarily neurological event as a rise in troponin can occur in subarachnoid haemorrhage. This patient did indeed have a subarachnoid haemorrhage, and the ECG eventually returned to normal.

> **SUMMARY**
>
> Anterolateral T wave inversion due to subarachnoid haemorrhage.

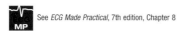 See *ECG Made Practical*, 7th edition, Chapter 8

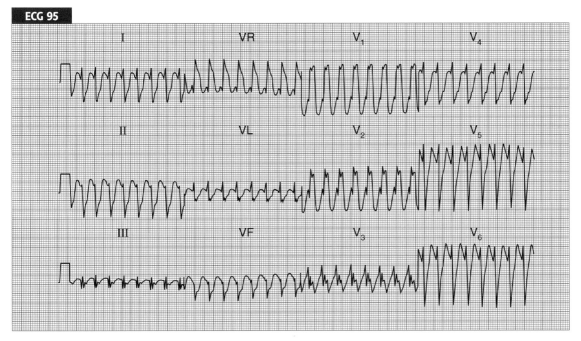

A 35-year-old woman, who had had palpitations for many years without any diagnosis being made, was eventually seen in the A&E department during an attack. She looked well and was not in heart failure, and her blood pressure was 120/70. This is her ECG. What is the rhythm, and what would you do?

ANSWER 95

The ECG shows:
- Broad complex tachycardia (QRS complex duration 200 ms), rate nearly 200 bpm
- No P waves visible
- Right axis deviation
- In lead V_1, the R^1 peak is higher than the R peak
- Right bundle branch block (RBBB) pattern
- No concordance of QRS complexes in the V leads.

Clinical interpretation

The problem here is to distinguish between a supraventricular tachycardia with bundle branch block and a ventricular tachycardia. The clinical history is not helpful, nor is the fact that the patient is haemodynamically stable. The combination of right axis deviation, RBBB and the R^1 peak being higher than the R peak in lead V_1 make it likely that this is a supraventricular tachycardia with RBBB rather than ventricular tachycardia. However, the very broad QRS complex (> 140 ms) would favour a ventricular origin for the arrhythmia.

What to do

Carotid sinus massage. If this has no effect, try intravenous adenosine. Cardioversion may be necessary.

SUMMARY

Broad complex tachycardia with RBBB pattern, probably supraventricular in origin.

 See *ECG Made Practical*, 7th edition, Chapter 4

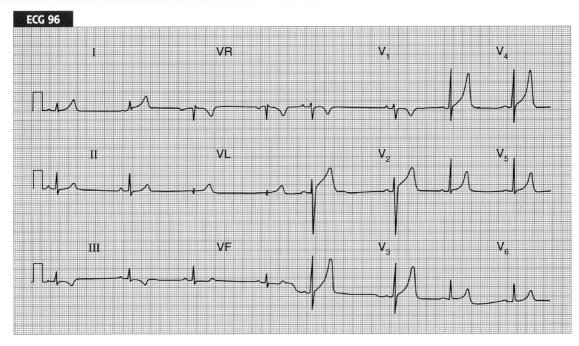

This ECG was recorded from a 37-year-old man admitted to hospital for a routine orthopaedic operation. The anaesthetist asks for comments.

ANSWER 96

The ECG shows:
- Sinus rhythm, average 45 bpm
- Normal axis
- Normal QRS complexes
- ST segment depression in lead VF
- Inverted T waves in leads III, VR, V_1
- Peaked T waves in the anterior leads.

Clinical interpretation

Provided the patient is not taking a beta-blocker, the slow heart rate is probably a reflection of physical fitness. Inverted T waves in leads III, VR and V_1, and the depressed ST segments in lead VF, are probably normal. Peaked T waves are characteristic of hyperkalaemia, and are sometimes described as 'hyperacute' in ischaemia. However, when as large as this – and particularly when the patient is asymptomatic – peaked T waves are nearly always perfectly normal.

What to do

Ensure that the patient has no cardiac symptoms, and check his electrolyte levels preoperatively.

> **SUMMARY**
>
> Normal ECG.

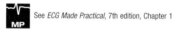 See *ECG Made Practical*, 7th edition, Chapter 1

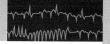

ECG 97

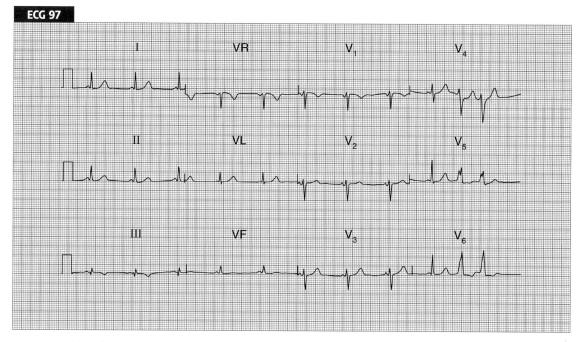

An 18-year-old student complains of occasional attacks of palpitations. These start suddenly without provocation; the heartbeat seems regular and is 'too fast to count'. During attacks she does not feel dizzy or breathless, and the palpitations stop suddenly after a few seconds. Physical examination is normal, and this is her ECG. What abnormalities on the ECG might be relevant, and what further test might be useful?

ANSWER 97

The ECG shows:

- Sinus rhythm, rate 64 bpm
- Very short PR interval
- The last two beats are extrasystoles. These could be ventricular, or atrial extrasystoles with a slurred upstroke due to aberrant conduction.
- Normal axis
- Small Q wave and inverted T wave in lead III (probably normal).

Clinical interpretation

There are two possible explanations for this patient's palpitations. The short PR interval might suggest an abnormal pathway but a slurred upstroke of the QRS which characterizes the Wolff–Parkinson–White (WPW) syndrome is not clearly seen in the sinus beats. Alternatively, the palpitations could be due to extrasystoles. An adenosine test may help to reveal an accessory pathway. Ambulatory monitoring may be required to make a definitive diagnosis.

What to do

An ECG recorded during symptoms is always the key to the diagnosis of palpitations, and some form of ambulatory monitoring should help. If a supraventricular tachycardia is detected an adenosine test might demonstrate an abnormal pathway, for adenosine will selectively block the atrioventricular node. An abnormal pathway might be amenable to ablation.

SUMMARY

Possible pre-excitation.

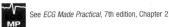 See *ECG Made Practical*, 7th edition, Chapter 2

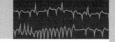

ECG 98

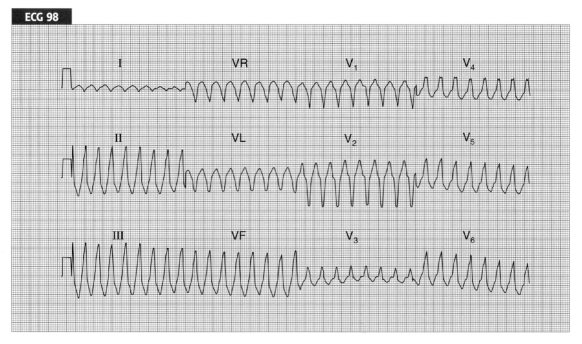

A 30-year-old man, who had had attacks of palpitations for several years, was seen during an attack, and this ECG was recorded. He was breathless and his blood pressure was unrecordable. What does the ECG show, and how should he be treated?

ANSWER 98

The ECG shows:
- Broad complex tachycardia at 200 bpm
- No P waves visible
- Right axis deviation
- QRS complex duration 200 ms
- QRS complexes show no concordance
- Left bundle branch block (LBBB) pattern – QRS complexes show 'M' pattern, best seen in lead V_4.

Clinical interpretation

A broad complex tachycardia like this is probably of ventricular origin. In this case, features against the rhythm being ventricular tachycardia are the right axis deviation and the lack of concordance in the QRS complexes (i.e. the complexes point downwards in leads V_1–V_2 and upwards in the other chest leads). The combination of right axis deviation and an LBBB pattern in a broad complex tachycardia suggests that the origin is in the right ventricular outflow tract.

What to do

Any patient with an arrhythmia and evidence of haemodynamic compromise (in this case, breathlessness and a very low blood pressure) needs immediate cardioversion. Once the arrhythmia has been corrected, an electrophysiological study is needed, because right ventricular outflow tract tachycardia is the one variety of ventricular tachycardia that should be amenable to ablation therapy.

SUMMARY

Ventricular tachycardia, probably originating in the right ventricular outflow tract.

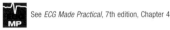 See *ECG Made Practical*, 7th edition, Chapter 4

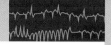

ECG 99

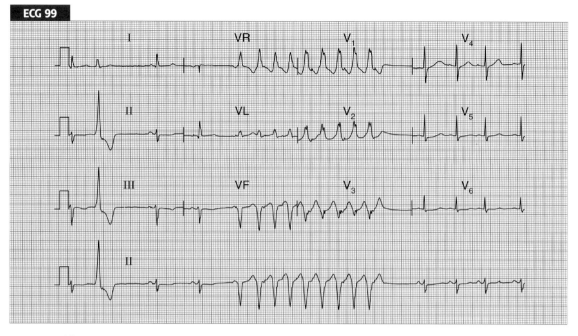

A 70-year-old man is sent to the outpatient department because of attacks of dizziness. What abnormalities does his ECG show, and what treatment is needed?

ANSWER 99

This ECG looks difficult to interpret because there is a nine-beat run of a broad complex tachycardia which occupies the whole of leads V_1–V_3. The key is to identify the rhythm first, from the lead II rhythm strip at the bottom. The ECG shows:

- The rhythm is basically sinus, with a rate varying between 65 bpm and 100 bpm
- One ventricular extrasystole, at the beginning of the record
- Broad complex tachycardia with an obviously different morphology from the sinus beats. The QRS complex duration is 160 ms, and in lead V_1 the R peak is higher that the R^1 peak. These features make it likely that the tachycardia is ventricular in origin
- Left axis deviation in the sinus beats (left anterior hemiblock)
- QRS complexes in the sinus beats otherwise appear normal
- Slight ST segment depression in leads II, III, V_5–V_6
- T wave inversion in leads II, III.

Clinical interpretation

This ECG shows paroxysmal ventricular tachycardia, and probably underlying ischaemic disease.

What to do

This patient's attacks of dizziness may be due to the paroxysmal arrhythmia, which is potentially life-threatening. The patient required further investigation including assessment of left ventricular systolic function (by echocardiography or cardiac MRI) and investigation for underlying coronary artery disease. Cautious introduction of a cardioselective betablocker may help to suppress further arrhythmia while definitive investigations are carried out.

SUMMARY

Sinus rhythm with paroxysmal ventricular tachycardia, and probable ischaemia.

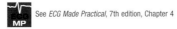 See *ECG Made Practical*, 7th edition, Chapter 4

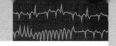

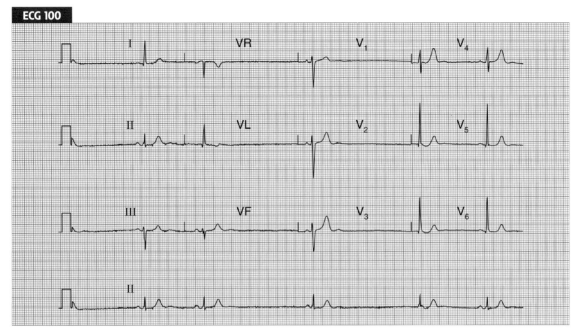

This is the ECG from a 25-year-old man who complained of episodes of fast, regular, palpitations associated with breathlessness and dizziness. There were no abnormalities on examination other than a slow and irregular pulse. What is the diagnosis and how can his problem be treated?

ANSWER 100

The ECG shows:
- Variable QRS complex rate, average 31 bpm
- Normal P waves in the first three beats; in the fourth beat the P wave immediately follows the QRS complex
- Normal QRS complexes and T waves

Clinical interpretation

This is the 'sick sinus syndrome' or 'sinoatrial disease'. The record shows sinus rhythm with a junctional escape beat, in which the atrium is activated retrogradely. The palpitations described by the patient are probably due to a paroxysmal supraventricular tachycardia, so he probably has the 'bradycardia–tachycardia' variant of sinoatrial disease.

What to do

Ambulatory ECG recording will confirm the cause of the patient's palpitations. Treatment will depend on the findings. His bradycardia does not require specific treatment unless he is symptomatic and permanent pacing should certainly be avoided unless absolutely essential given his age.

> **SUMMARY**
>
> Sinoatrial disease with sinus rhythm and a junctional escape beat.

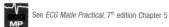 See *ECG Made Practical*, 7th edition Chapter 5

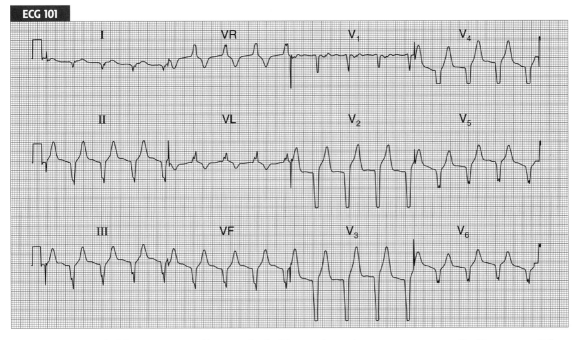

This ECG was recorded from a 45-year-old man, who had been admitted to a coronary care unit with a myocardial infarction and who was recovering well. What is the rhythm, and what would you do?

ANSWER 101

The ECG shows:
- Broad complex rhythm, rate 90 bpm
- No P waves
- Marked left axis deviation
- QRS complex duration 160 ms
- All chest leads show a downward QRS complex (concordance).

Clinical interpretation

If the heart rate were fast there would be little difficulty in recognizing this as ventricular tachycardia, and this rhythm used to be called 'slow VT'. It is, however, an accelerated idioventricular rhythm.

What to do

This rhythm is quite commonly seen in patients with an acute myocardial infarction, particularly following reperfusion, and indeed is not uncommon in ambulatory ECG records from normal people. It never causes problems, and it is important not to attempt to treat it: suppressing any 'escape' rhythm may lead to a dangerous bradycardia.

SUMMARY

Accelerated idioventricular rhythm.

 See *ECG Made Practical*, 7th edition, Chapter 1

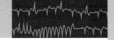

ECG 102

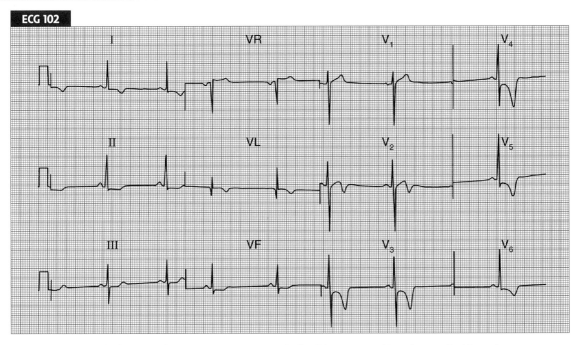

This ECG was recorded as part of a routine examination of a healthy 25-year-old professional athlete. There were no abnormal physical findings. What does it show and what would you do?

ANSWER 102

The ECG shows:
- Sinus rhythm, average rate 44 bpm
- Normal axis
- Normal QRS complexes, apart from narrow Q waves in lead VL
- Marked T wave inversion in leads I, VL, V_2–V_6.

Clinical interpretation

If this ECG had been recorded from a middle-aged man presenting with acute chest pain, the diagnosis would be an anterior non-ST segment elevation myocardial infarction. The ECGs of athletes can show ST segment and T wave changes due to left ventricular hypertrophy, but anteroseptal T wave inversion of this degree in a healthy young man almost certainly represents hypertrophic cardiomyopathy.

What to do

Echocardiography will confirm the diagnosis. Ambulatory ECG recording will show whether the patient is having ventricular arrhythmias. If the diagnosis is confirmed, he should be counselled not to play competitive sports. He should be referred for genetic testing and his close relatives should be screened.

> **SUMMARY**
>
> Probable hypertrophic cardiomyopathy.

 See *ECG Made Practical*, 7th edition, Chapter 3

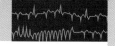

ECG 103

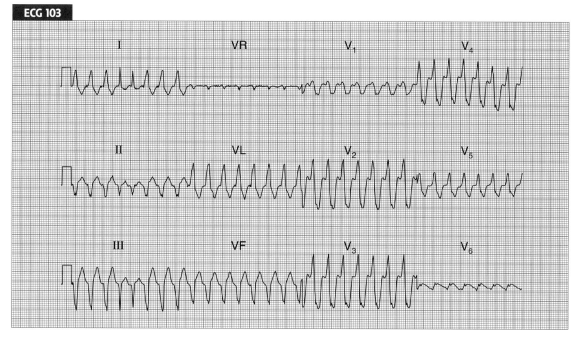

A 70-year-old woman, admitted to hospital because of increasing heart failure of uncertain cause, collapsed and was found to have a very rapid pulse and a low blood pressure. This is her ECG. She recovered spontaneously. What is this rhythm, and what would you do?

ANSWER 103

The ECG shows:

- Broad complex tachycardia at about 188 bpm
- No P waves visible
- Left axis deviation
- QRS complex duration about 140 ms
- Narrow fourth and fifth QRS complexes
- QRS complexes that are probably concordant (in the chest leads all point upwards) though it is difficult to be certain.

Clinical interpretation

Broad complex tachycardias may be ventricular, supraventricular with bundle branch block, or due to the Wolff–Parkinson–White syndrome. We have no ECG from this patient recorded in sinus rhythm, which is always the most helpful thing in deciding between these possibilities. The complexes are not very wide, which would be consistent with a supraventricular origin with aberrant conduction, but the left axis deviation and (probable) concordance point to ventricular tachycardia. The key is the two narrow complexes near the beginning of the record: these are slightly early and are probably capture beats. They indicate that with an early supraventricular beat the conducting system can function normally; by implication, the broad complexes must be due to ventricular tachycardia.

What to do

In the first instance restoration of sinus rhythm by DC cardioversion under sedation or anaesthesia is indicated. An older patient with heart failure is more likely to have ischaemic disease than anything else, but all the possible causes of heart failure must be considered. The sudden onset of an arrhythmia could also be due to a myocardial infarction which should be evident on the post-cardioversion ECG. It is important to consider whether this rhythm change is related to treatment, in which case it could be due to an electrolyte imbalance or to the pro-arrhythmic effect of a drug the patient is taking.

SUMMARY

Ventricular tachycardia.

 See *ECG Made Practical*, 7th edition, Chapter 4

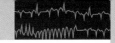

ECG 104

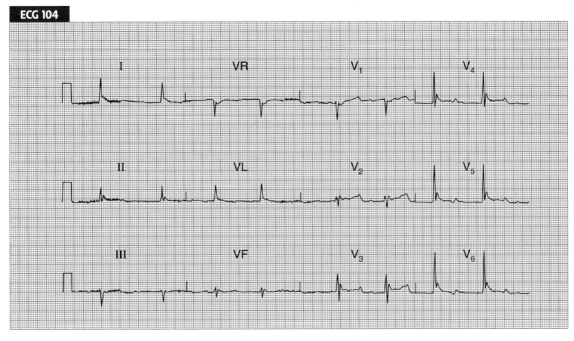

This ECG was recorded from an 80-year-old woman who had been found unconscious with physical signs suggesting a stroke. Any comments?

ANSWER 104

The ECG shows:
- Atrial fibrillation with a ventricular rate of about 55 bpm
- QRS complex duration prolonged at 200 ms
- Prominent 'J' waves, best seen in leads V_3–V_6
- Widespread but nonspecific ST segment/T wave changes.

Clinical interpretation

The atrial fibrillation may or may not be related to her stroke – she may have had a cerebral embolus, or she may have both coronary and cerebrovascular disease. The slow ventricular rate and the 'J' waves indicate hypothermia, and her core temperature was 25°C. ECGs from hypothermic patients seldom show 'J' waves as clearly as this because there are too many artefacts due to shivering – but this patient was too cold to shiver. She did not survive.

> **SUMMARY**
>
> Atrial fibrillation and hypothermia.

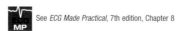 See *ECG Made Practical*, 7th edition, Chapter 8

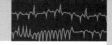

ECG 105

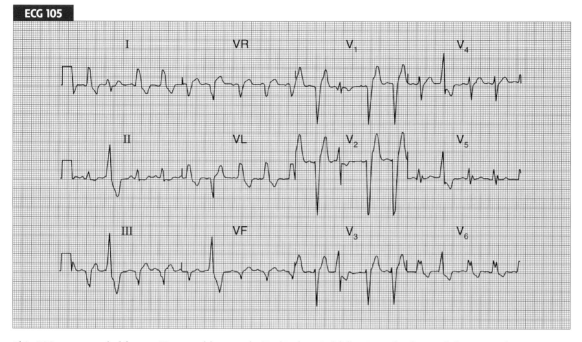

This ECG was recorded from a 50-year-old man admitted to hospital following 2 h of central chest pain that was characteristic of a myocardial infarction. His ECG had been normal 6 months ago. What does this record show and what would you do?

ANSWER 105

The ECG shows:
- Sinus rhythm, rate about 107 bpm
- Ventricular extrasystoles
- Normal axis
- Wide QRS complexes, with 'M' pattern in lead V_6, and inverted T waves in leads I, VL, V_5–V_6 – indicating left bundle branch block (LBBB) in the sinus beats.

Clinical interpretation

The ventricular extrasystoles can be identified because they have a different morphology from the LBBB pattern, and because they have no preceding P waves. LBBB masks any changes there might be as the result of a myocardial infarction.

What to do

The LBBB has evidently developed in the last 6 months, and the history suggests a myocardial infarction and the patient should be managed accordingly with dual antiplatelet therapy (aspirin and a P2Y12 inhibitor) and emergency angiography with a view to primary angioplasty. The ventricular extrasystoles do not require specific treatment.

> **SUMMARY**
>
> Sinus rhythm with LBBB and ventricular extrasystoles.

 See *ECG Made Practical*, 7th edition, Chapter 6

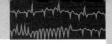

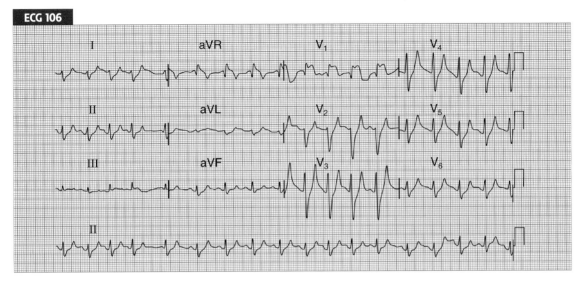

A 75-year-old woman was admitted with heart failure. She had been treated with digoxin, ramipril, Frumil and Spironolactone. Does her ECG suggest any particular problems?

ANSWER 106

The ECG shows:
- Sinus rhythm with atrial extrasystoles, rate 100 bpm
- Right axis deviation
- Broad QRS (140 ms) with right bundle branch block (RBBB) pattern
- Symmetrically peaked T waves.

Clinical interpretation

Potentially the most important abnormality is the peaking of the T waves, which suggests hyperkalaemia. Her medication – an angiotensin-converting enzyme inhibitor, Frumil (which contains amiloride), and spironolactone – would be a potent cause of hyperkalaemia, and this was the case here. The RBBB might or might not be new, and earlier ECGs would be helpful.

What to do

Stop the potassium-retaining drugs (Frumil and, particularly, spironolactone). Measure the serum potassium and treat hyperkalaemia accordingly. Intravenous calcium carbonate/calcium gluoconate together with insulin dextrose and nebulized salbutamol may be required if severe but check and follow your local management guidelines.

SUMMARY

Hyperkalaemia and RBBB.

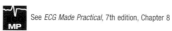 See *ECG Made Practical*, 7th edition, Chapter 8

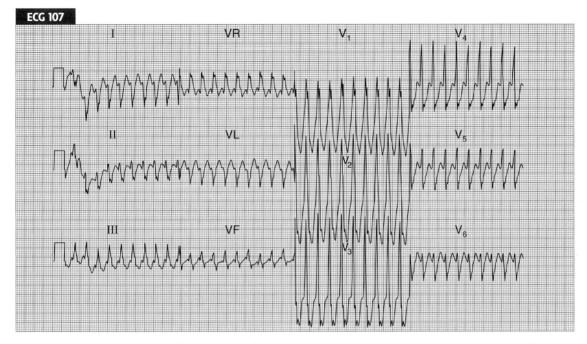

A 30-year-old man, who had had brief episodes of palpitations for at least 10 years, was seen during an attack in the A&E department and this is his ECG. What is the rhythm, and what would you do immediately, and in the long term?

ANSWER 107

The ECG shows:
- Broad complex tachycardia at about 230–240 bpm
- No P waves visible
- Right axis deviation
- QRS complex duration of about 180 ms
- QRS complexes point upwards in lead V_1 and downwards in lead V_6 – no concordance
- QRS complex configuration characteristic of right bundle branch block – but in lead V_1 the first R wave peak is higher than the second peak.

Clinical interpretation

There are essentially three causes of a broad complex tachycardia: ventricular tachycardia, supraventricular tachycardia with bundle branch block and the Wolff–Parkinson–White (WPW) syndrome. The key to the diagnosis lies in the ECG when the heart is in sinus rhythm, but this is not always available. Patients with a broad complex tachycardia in the context of an acute myocardial infarction must be assumed to have a ventricular tachycardia, but that does not apply here. In this record, the QRS complexes are not very broad, the axis is to the right, and there is no concordance of the QRS complexes – all pointing to a supraventricular origin. In favour of a ventricular tachycardia is the fact that the height of the primary R wave in lead V_1 is greater than that of the secondary R wave. However, taking these features together with the clinical picture, the rhythm is probably supraventricular.

What to do

Carotid sinus pressure or adenosine is a reasonable first move. If there is severe haemodynamic compromise the patient may need urgent electrical cardioversion. In fact, in this case the arrhythmia terminated spontaneously, revealing a short PR interval and a QRS complex with a delta wave. So this patient had the WPW syndrome, and needed an electrophysiological study with a view to ablation of the accessory tract.

SUMMARY

Broad complex tachycardia (eventually shown to be due to the WPW syndrome).

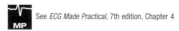 See *ECG Made Practical*, 7th edition, Chapter 4

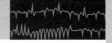

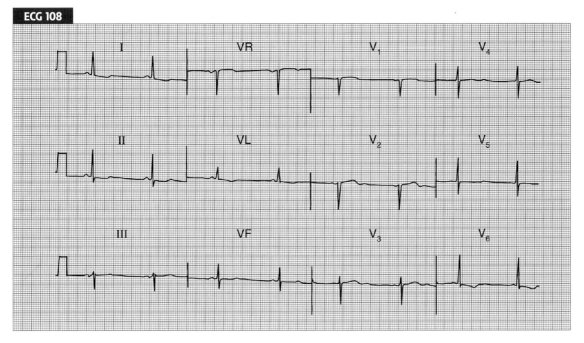

This ECG was recorded as part of a routine health check on a 50-year-old woman who said she was asymptomatic. The only abnormality detected in the other usual screening tests was a serum cholesterol level of 7.2 mmol/l. What would you do?

ANSWER 108

The ECG shows:
- Sinus rhythm, rate 45 bpm
- Normal axis
- Normal QRS complexes
- Widespread T wave flattening and inversion
- Prominent U waves, especially in leads V_2–V_5.

Clinical interpretation

Flattened T waves with prominent U waves usually result from hypokalaemia. The serum potassium level is usually checked during health screening, but the same ECG changes can result from hypomagnesaemia; hypocalcaemia causes a long QT interval but not U waves. A high cholesterol level can be a marker for coronary disease, but elevated cholesterol levels can also be secondary to thyroid or renal disease.

What to do

Check a full blood screen. In this case the answer came from the thyroid function tests. This woman had myxoedema, and her ECG became normal when it was treated.

SUMMARY

Widespread T wave flattening with prominent U waves – classically due to hypokalaemia, but in this case due to myxoedema.

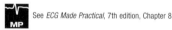 See *ECG Made Practical*, 7th edition, Chapter 8

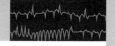

ECG 109

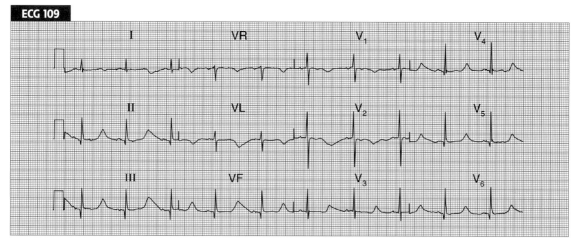

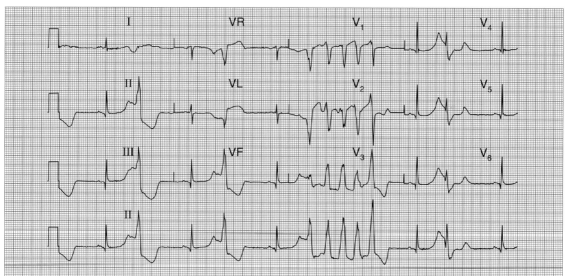

A confused 80-year-old woman was sent to hospital from a nursing home because of a collapse. No other history was available, except that she was said to be having treatment for her heart. There were no obvious physical signs. The upper ECG was recorded on admission, and the lower ECG was recorded shortly afterwards. What is going on?

ANSWER 109

The upper ECG shows:
- Sinus rhythm, with a rate of 60 bpm
- Narrow Q waves in leads II, III, VF, V_4–V_6
- Abnormally shaped T waves in most leads
- Prolonged QT interval (about 650 ms).

The lower ECG shows:
- Sinus rhythm with multifocal ventricular extrasystoles
- A run of polymorphic (i.e. changing shape) ventricular tachycardia.

Clinical interpretation

In the upper trace the inferolateral Q waves could represent an old infarction, but they are narrow and are probably septal in origin. The prolonged QT interval and abnormal T waves suggest either an electrolyte abnormality or that the patient is being treated with one of the many drugs that have these effects. A collapse in a patient with an ECG with a long QT interval suggests episodes of torsade de pointes ventricular tachycardia.

What to do

The electrolyte levels, including magnesium, must be checked, and in this case were found to be normal. It is essential immediately to establish what medication the patient is taking, and pending that information it would be sensible to leave her untreated and simply to monitor her for arrhythmias. It turned out that this woman was taking sotalol – a beta-blocker with class III antiarrhythmic activity which is known to cause QT interval prolongation. When this drug was stopped, her ECG returned to normal.

SUMMARY

Drug-induced QT interval prolongation and polymorphic ventricular tachycardia.

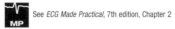 See *ECG Made Practical*, 7th edition, Chapter 2

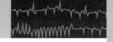

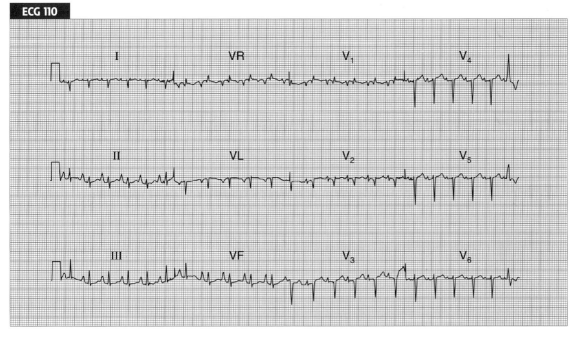

This ECG was recorded from a 60-year-old man seen in the clinic because of severe breathlessness, which had developed over several years. His jugular venous pressure is raised. What do you think is the problem?

ANSWER 110

The ECG shows:

- Sinus rhythm, rate 140 bpm
- One ventricular extrasystole
- Peaked P waves (best seen in leads II, III, VF)
- Normal PR interval
- Right axis deviation
- Dominant R wave in lead V_1
- Deep S wave in lead V_6
- Normal ST segments and T waves.

Clinical interpretation

The sinus tachycardia suggests a major problem. The peaked P waves indicate right atrial hypertrophy. The right axis deviation and dominant R wave in lead V_1 suggest right ventricular hypertrophy. The deep S wave in lead V_6, with no 'left ventricular' complexes in the chest leads, indicates 'clockwise rotation' of the heart, with the right ventricle occupying the precordium. These changes suggest lung disease.

What to do

Since the ECG is entirely 'right-sided', one can assume that the problem is due to chronic lung disease or recurrent pulmonary embolism. The story sounds more in keeping with a lung problem. The raised jugular venous pressure is presumably due to cor pulmonale. The sinus tachycardia is worrying, and suggests respiratory failure.

SUMMARY

Sinus tachycardia and one ventricular extrasystole; right atrial and right ventricular hypertrophy; and clockwise rotation – suggesting chronic lung disease.

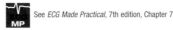 See *ECG Made Practical*, 7th edition, Chapter 7

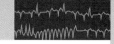

ECG 111

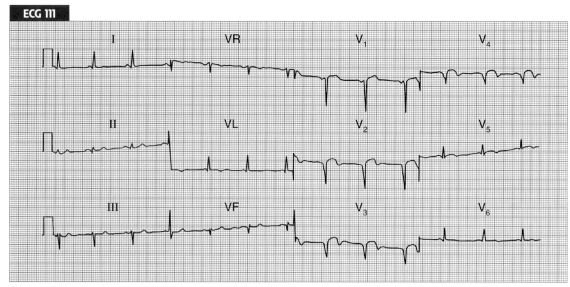

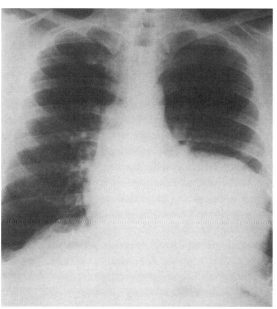

A 60-year-old man is seen in the outpatient department complaining of breathlessness which began quite suddenly 2 months previously. He had had no chest pain. Examination revealed a raised jugular venous pressure, basal crackles in the lungs and a third sound at the cardiac apex. These are his ECG and chest X-ray. What do they show, and how does this fit the clinical picture? What would you do?

ANSWER 111

The ECG shows:
- Sinus rhythm, rate 72 bpm
- Normal axis
- Large Q waves in leads V_1–V_4 and small Q waves in leads I, VL
- Elevated ST segments and inverted T waves in leads V_2–V_5
- Flattened T waves in leads I and V_6; inverted T waves in lead VL.

The chest X-ray shows a left ventricular aneurysm.

Clinical interpretation

This ECG would be compatible with an acute anterior myocardial infarction, but this does not fit the clinical picture: it appears that an event occurred 2 months previously. This pattern of ST segment elevation in the anterior leads can persist following a large infarction, and is often seen in the presence of a ventricular aneurysm. This is confirmed by the chest X-ray.

What to do

An echocardiogram will show the extent of the aneurysm and whether the remaining left ventricular function is impaired, which it almost certainly will be. Further investigations will be required to assess the underlying coronary artery disease and the extent of myocardial viability. The patient should be treated with guideline-based treatment for heart failure and ischaemic heart disease.

> **SUMMARY**
>
> Old anterior myocardial infarction with a left ventricular aneurysm.

 See *ECG Made Practical*, 7th edition, Chapter 7

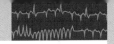

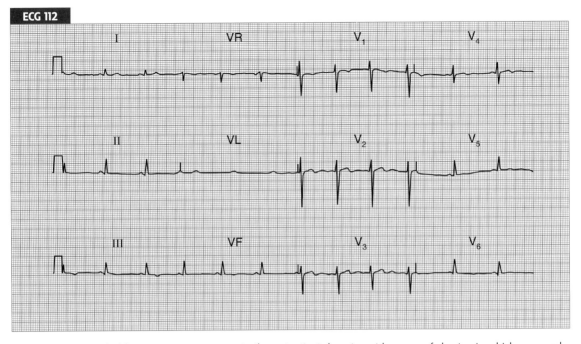

This ECG was recorded from a young man seen in the outpatient department because of chest pain which appeared to be nonspecific. How would you interpret the ECG, and what action would you take?

ANSWER 112

The ECG shows:

- Sinus rhythm, rate 71 bpm
- Normal axis
- Normal QRS complexes
- Inverted T waves in leads III, VF; biphasic T waves in lead V_4; flattened T waves in leads V_5–V_6
- U waves in leads V_2–V_3 (normal).

Clinical interpretation

These T wave changes, particularly those in the inferior leads, could well be caused by ischaemia. The flattened T waves in the lateral leads can only be described as 'nonspecific'.

What to do

When confronted with an ECG showing this sort of 'nonspecific' abnormality, action depends primarily on the clinical diagnosis. If the patient is asymptomatic it is fair to report the ECG as showing 'nonspecific changes'; if the patient has symptoms at all – as in this case – it is probably worth proceeding to further investigations. In this case CT coronary angiography was normal. A repeat ECG, recorded purely out of interest a month later, showed similar changes.

> **SUMMARY**
>
> Nonspecific ST segment and T wave changes.

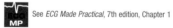 See *ECG Made Practical*, 7th edition, Chapter 1

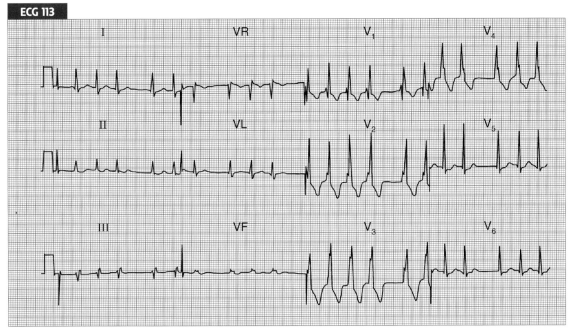

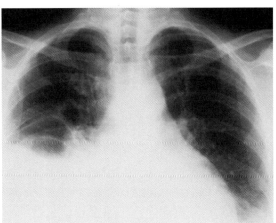

A 60-year-old man, whose heart and preoperative ECG had been normal, developed a cough with pleuritic chest pain a few days after a cholecystectomy. These are his ECG and chest X-ray: what do they show and what might be the problem?

ANSWER 113

The ECG shows:
- Atrial fibrillation
- Normal axis
- RSR^1 pattern in leads V$_1$–V$_3$, indicating right bundle branch block (RBBB).

The chest X-ray shows a large pleural effusion on the right side with some atelectasis above it, and also a small left-sided effusion. There is upper-zone blood diversion, indicating heart failure.

Clinical interpretation

In this ECG the usual 'irregular baseline' of atrial fibrillation is not apparent, but the QRS complexes are so irregular that this must be the rhythm. The rhythm change, together with the development of RBBB, could be due to a chest infection but is more likely to have been caused by a pulmonary embolus. The right-sided pleural effusion could also be due to either infection or embolism, but the patient clearly has heart failure because the effusions are bilateral (although asymmetrical) and there is diversion of blood flow to the upper zones of the lungs.

What to do

In a postoperative patient, anticoagulation does not usually cause haemorrhage once postoperative haemostasis has been achieved, however full multidisciplinary discussion with the surgical team is sensible. Nevertheless, the risk of death from a pulmonary embolus is so high that the patient should be given low molecular weight heparin while steps are taken (white blood cell count, computed tomography pulmonary angiography) to differentiate between a chest infection and a pulmonary embolus.

SUMMARY

Atrial fibrillation with RBBB.

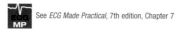 See *ECG Made Practical*, 7th edition, Chapter 7

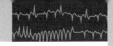

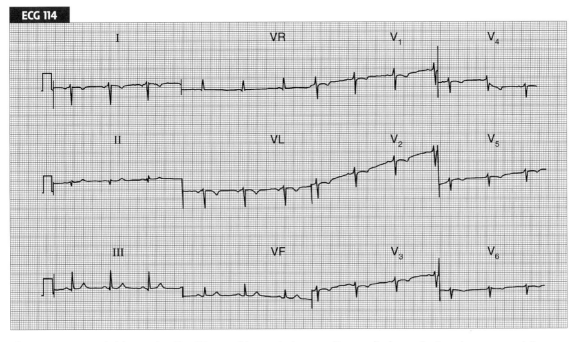

This ECG was recorded from a healthy 25-year-old man during a routine medical examination. Any comments?

ANSWER 114

The ECG shows:
- A very odd appearance
- Sinus rhythm, rate 70 bpm
- Inverted P waves in lead I
- Right axis deviation
- Dominant R waves in lead VR
- No R wave development in the chest leads, with lead V_6 still showing a right ventricular pattern
- Normal-width QRS complexes.

Clinical interpretation

This is dextrocardia. A normal trace would be obtained with the limb leads reversed and the chest leads attached in the usual rib spaces but on the right side of the chest.

What to do

Ensure that the leads are properly attached – for example, inverted P waves in lead I will be seen if the right and left arm attachments are reversed. Of course, this would not affect the appearance of the ECG in the chest leads.

SUMMARY

Dextrocardia.

 See *ECG Made Practical*, 7th edition, Chapter 1

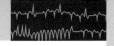

ECG 115

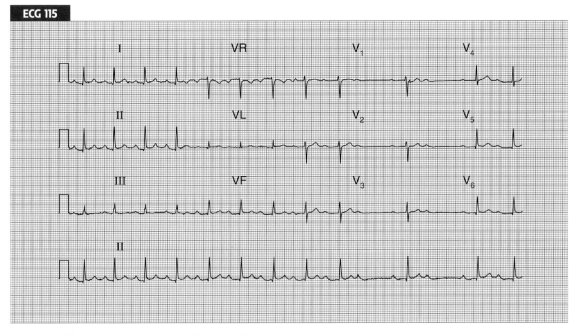

A 70-year-old man with long-standing high blood pressure has had attacks of dizziness over several weeks. His pulse feels irregular, but there are no other abnormal signs. This was his ECG. What does it show, and what would you do?

ANSWER 115

The ECG shows:
- The first nine beats with sinus rhythm and a ventricular rate of about 80 bpm
- The PR interval in these nine beats slowly increases, from 240 to 360 ms
- There is then a nonconducted P wave, followed by a conducted P wave with a PR interval of 360 ms
- There is then a second nonconducted P wave, followed by two conducted P waves, again with a PR interval of 360 ms
- Normal axis
- Normal QRS complexes, ST segments and T waves.

Clinical interpretation

This ECG shows a mixture of different types of heart block. The progressively increasing PR intervals followed by a nonconducted P wave represent second degree block of the Wenckebach (Mobitz type 1) type. The next nonconducted P wave followed by a conducted P wave with a long PR interval is second degree block of Mobitz type 2. The final beat, with the same prolonged PR interval, shows first degree block. The changing heart rate is presumably the cause of his attacks of dizziness.

What to do

Although this man has had no pain, and there is no evidence of ischaemia on the ECG, coronary disease may still be responsible for the conduction problem, but in a hypertensive patient one potential contribution to this sort of heart block is medication. He may well be taking either a beta-blocker or a calcium-blocker, and the first thing to do would be to discontinue these and then reassess symptoms and ambulatory ECG monitoring before making a final decision as to whether permanent pacing is indicated.

> **SUMMARY**
>
> Second degree block of both the Wenckebach type and Mobitz type 2, and also first degree block.

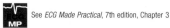 See *ECG Made Practical*, 7th edition, Chapter 3

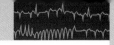

ECG 116

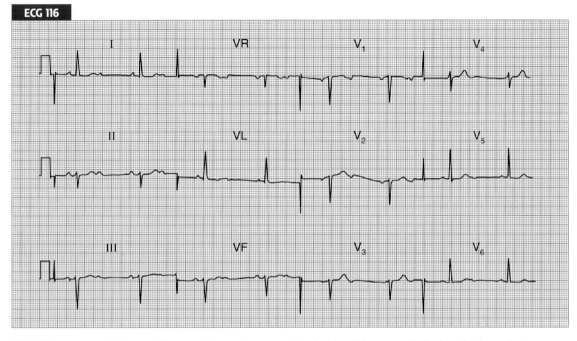

This ECG was recorded from a 75-year-old man who complained of breathlessness. He had not had any chest pain or dizziness. Apart from a slow pulse, there were no abnormalities on examination. What three abnormalities are present in this record, and how would you treat the patient?

ANSWER 116

The ECG shows:
- Sinus rhythm; ventricular rate 45 bpm
- Second degree (2:1) block
- Left axis deviation
- Poor R wave progression in the anterior leads
- Normal T waves.

Clinical interpretation

The second degree block is associated with a ventricular rate of 45 bpm, which may well be the cause of his breathlessness. The left axis deviation indicates left anterior hemiblock. The poor R wave progression (virtually no R wave in lead V_3, a small R wave in lead V_4 and a normal R wave in lead V_5) suggests an old anterior infarction.

What to do

This patient needs a permanent pacemaker.

SUMMARY

Second degree (2:1) block, left anterior hemiblock and probable old anterior infarction.

 See *ECG Made Practical*, 7th edition, Chapter 5

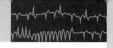

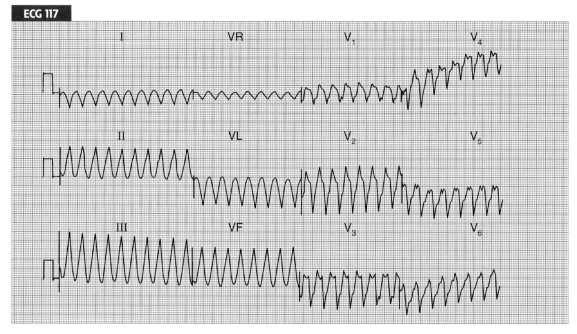

This ECG was recorded in a coronary care unit from a patient admitted 2 h previously with an acute anterior myocardial infarction. The patient was cold, clammy and confused, and his blood pressure was unrecordable. What does the ECG show, and what would you do?

ANSWER 117

The ECG shows:

- Broad complex tachycardia, rate about 215 bpm
- Regular QRS complexes
- QRS complex duration uncertain: probably about 280 ms
- Indeterminate axis and QRS complex configuration.

Clinical interpretation

In the context of acute myocardial infarction, broad complex tachycardias should be considered to be ventricular in origin – unless the patient is known to have bundle branch block when in sinus rhythm. Here, the regularity of the rhythm and the very broad complexes of bizarre configuration leave no room for doubt that this is ventricular tachycardia.

What to do

In cases of severe circulatory failure, immediate direct current (DC) cardioversion is needed.

SUMMARY

Ventricular tachycardia.

 See *ECG Made Practical*, 7th edition, Chapter 4

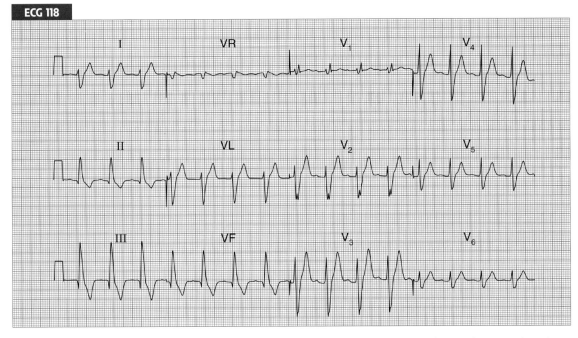

An 80-year-old woman complained of breathlessness and frequent attacks of dizziness. This was her ECG when she attended the clinic. What does the ECG show, what might the dizziness be due to, and how would you manage her?

ANSWER 118

The ECG shows:
- Sinus rhythm, rate 90 bpm
- Right axis deviation
- Right bundle branch block (RBBB).

Clinical interpretation

The right axis deviation suggests left posterior hemiblock, and, combined with RBBB, this suggests bifascicular block. The patient is therefore at risk of complete (third degree) block, which could cause a Stokes–Adams attack.

What to do

Ambulatory monitoring is required to confirm bradyarrhythmias. This woman was in fact admitted to hospital and monitored, and had a severe attack of dizziness and fainting. During this attack, another ECG was recorded (see below). This ECG shows complete heart block with a ventricular rate of about 15 bpm. The patient was immediately given a permanent pacemaker.

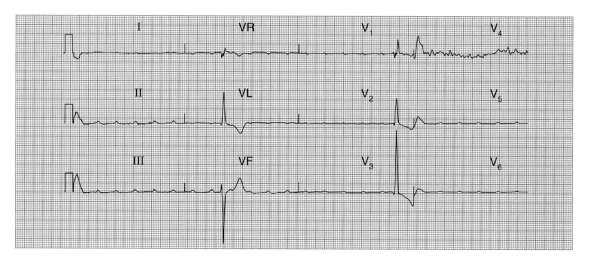

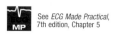
See *ECG Made Practical*,
7th edition, Chapter 5

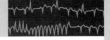

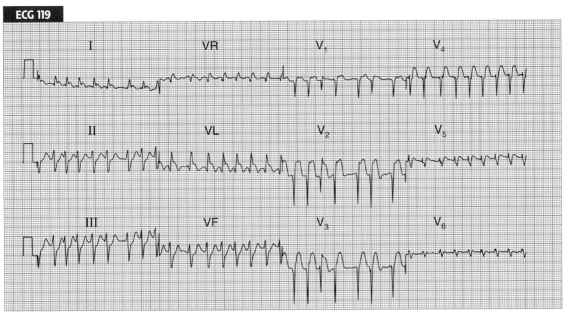

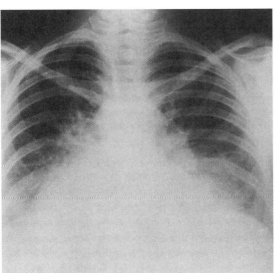

This ECG and chest X-ray were recorded from a diabetic man who was admitted to hospital because of the sudden onset of pulmonary oedema. What do you think has happened?

ANSWER 119

The ECG shows:

- Atrial fibrillation with a ventricular rate of about 180 bpm
- Left axis deviation
- Probable Q waves in leads V_2–V_4
- QRS complexes of normal width and height
- Raised ST segments in leads I, VL, V_2–V_4.

The chest X-ray shows pulmonary oedema; it is difficult to see the heart borders.

Clinical interpretation

This ECG shows uncontrolled atrial fibrillation with left anterior hemiblock and an acute anterolateral ST segment elevation myocardial infarction (STEMI). The onset of atrial fibrillation may have been a consequence of the myocardial infarction, and the rapid ventricular rate will at least in part explain the pulmonary oedema. The left anterior hemiblock is probably a consequence of the infarction. The patient may not have experienced pain because of his diabetes.

What to do

The most important thing is to relieve the patient's distress and the pulmonary oedema. He needs diamorphine and intravenous nitrates. Management of his tachyarrythmia is complicated by the risk that beta-blockers could worsen his pulmonary oedema. In this context intravenous amiodarone, digoxin or even DC cardioversion may be required. Attention can then be turned to the treatment of his myocardial infarction. He will need dual antiplatelet therapy and emergency angiography with a view to primary angioplasty.

> **SUMMARY**
>
> Atrial fibrillation, left anterior hemiblock and acute anterolateral STEMI.

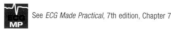 See *ECG Made Practical*, 7th edition, Chapter 7

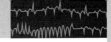

ECG 120

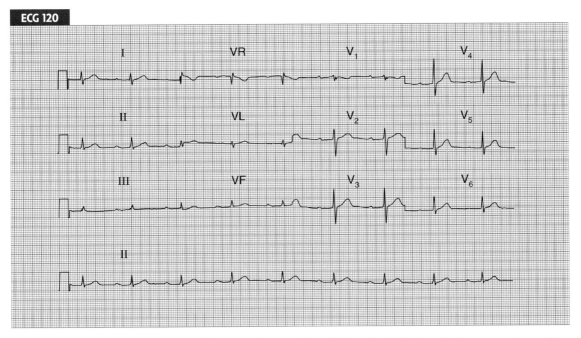

This ECG was recorded from a 75-year-old woman who complained of attacks of dizziness. It shows one abnormality: what is its significance?

ANSWER 120

The ECG shows:
- Sinus rhythm, 55 bpm
- Prolonged PR interval of 320 ms
- Normal axis
- RSR¹ pattern in lead V_1, with normal QRS complex duration: partial right bundle branch block (RBBB)
- Normal ST segments and T waves.

Clinical interpretation

Sinus rhythm with first degree block. The partial RBBB is probably not significant.

What to do

First degree block does not cause any haemodynamic impairment, and by itself is of little significance. However, when a patient has symptoms (in this case, dizziness) which might be due to a bradycardia, there may be episodes of second or third degree block, or possibly Stokes–Adams attacks, associated with a slow ventricular rate. The appropriate action is therefore to request an ambulatory ECG. The approach will depend on the frequency of symptoms with 24 hour monitoring suitable for frequent (more than once per day) episodes, with a loop recorder (including implantable devices) more suitable for less frequent symptoms. It would then be possible to see whether the dizziness was associated with a change in heart rhythm. First degree block itself is not an indication for permanent pacing or for any other intervention.

SUMMARY

Sinus rhythm with first degree block.

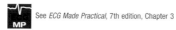 See *ECG Made Practical*, 7th edition, Chapter 3

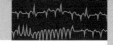

ECG 121

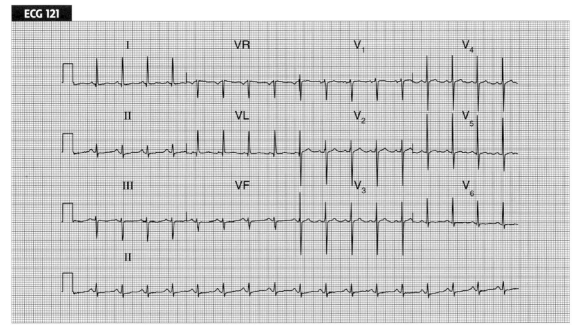

This ECG was recorded from a 35-year-old woman who complained of breathlessness but not of pain. She was anxious, but there were no abnormalities on examination. Does this ECG help with her diagnosis and management?

ANSWER 121

The ECG shows:
- Sinus rhythm, rate 106 bpm
- Normal axis
- Normal QRS complexes (septal Q waves in leads I and VL)
- Slight ST segment depression, especially in leads II and V_6
- T wave flattening in leads II, III, VF, V_6
- T wave inversion in lead III.

Clinical interpretation

A sinus rate of over 100 bpm would be compatible with anxiety, though other causes of 'high output' (e.g. pregnancy, thyrotoxicosis, anaemia, volume loss, CO_2 retention) have to be considered. The widespread ST segment and T wave changes have to be described as 'nonspecific'; in an anxious patient they could be due to hyperventilation. The ECG does not help with the diagnosis and management.

What to do

If a full history and examination fail to suggest any underlying physical disease, further investigations are unlikely to be helpful.

SUMMARY

Nonspecific ST segment and T wave changes.

 See *ECG Made Practical*, 7th edition, Chapter 1

ECG 122

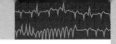

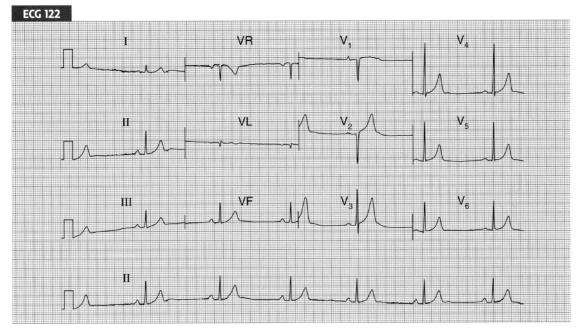

This ECG was recorded from a 40-year-old man who was well and ran marathons. Despite showing four possible 'abnormalities', is the trace actually normal?

ANSWER 122

The ECG shows:
- Sinus rhythm, average rate 39 bpm
- Bifid P waves, best seen in the anterior chest leads
- Normal axis
- QRS complexes show left ventricular hypertrophy on voltage criteria (R wave in lead V_4=25 mm)
- Peaked T waves.

Clinical interpretation

Sinus bradycardia can be due to physical fitness, vagal overactivity or myxoedema. In a hypertensive patient, beta-blocker treatment is a possible explanation. The bifid P waves may indicate left atrial hypertrophy ('P mitrale'), but can be normal. Voltage criteria for left ventricular hypertrophy are extremely unreliable when there is no other evidence of this. The peaked T waves could be due to hyperkalaemia but are more often a normal variant.

What to do

All these possible abnormalities are seen in normal athletes, and the likelihood is that they are of no significance.

SUMMARY

Normal ECG for an athlete.

 See *ECG Made Practical*, 7th edition, Chapter 1

ECG 123

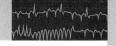

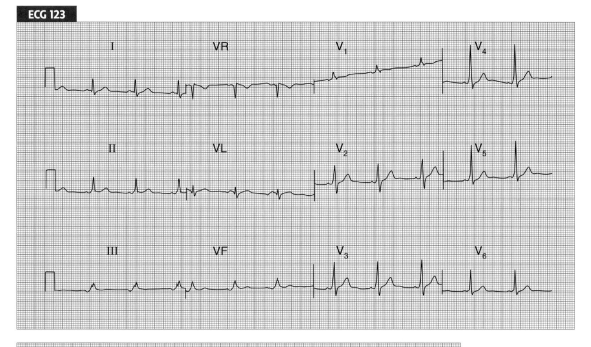

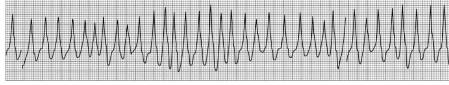

A 30-year-old woman complains of episodes of palpitations associated with dizziness and breathlessness. These begin and stop suddenly. She has had them for many years, but they are becoming more frequent and more severe. The upper ECG was recorded at rest; the lower ECG is part of an ambulatory record, during which she had a typical attack. What do these ECGs show and what would you do?

ANSWER 123

The upper ECG shows:
- Sinus rhythm, rate 64 bpm
- Short PR interval, best seen in leads V_4–V_5
- Normal axis
- Dominant R waves in lead V_1
- Slurred upstroke (delta wave) in the QRS complexes.

The lower ECG (rhythm strip) shows:
- A broad complex tachycardia
- Rate about 230 bpm
- The rhythm is irregular
- There is a slurred upstroke in some of the beats, suggesting pre-excitation.

Clinical interpretation

This is the Wolff–Parkinson–White (WPW) syndrome, involving a short PR interval and a widened QRS complex. This pattern, with a dominant R wave in lead V_1 and where there is a left-sided accessory pathway, is called 'type A'. It can easily be mistaken for right ventricular hypertrophy. The patient's palpitations are due to atrial fibrillation; an irregular broad complex tachycardia is characteristic of atrial fibrillation in the WPW syndrome.

What to do

Atrial fibrillation in association with the WPW syndrome is extremely dangerous. The patient should be treated with Flecainide pending an urgent electrophysiological study with a view to ablation of the accessory pathway. An ECG was recorded after the ablation (see right – leads V_4–V_6 shown): the PR interval is now normal and there is no widening of the QRS complex.

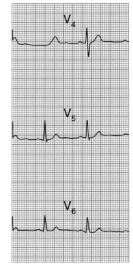

SUMMARY

The WPW syndrome type A, with paroxysmal atrial fibrillation.

See *ECG Made Practical*, 7th edition, Chapter 2

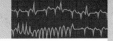

ECG 124

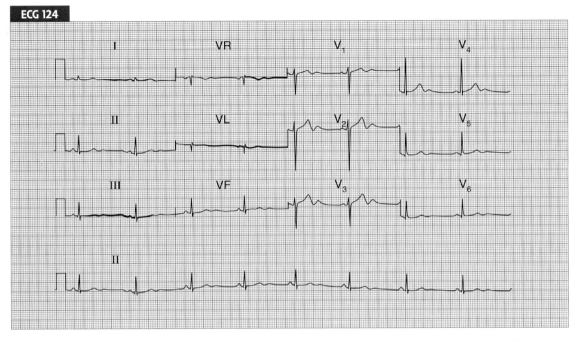

This ECG was recorded from a 30-year-old man at a medical examination required by the Civil Aviation Authority. Is it normal?

ANSWER 124

The ECG shows:
- Sinus rhythm, rate 52 bpm
- Prominent U waves, especially in leads V_2–V_4.

Clinical interpretation

U waves can indicate hypokalaemia, but when associated with normal T waves (as here) they are a normal variant.

What to do

Provide reassurance – on the basis of his ECG at least, he is fit to fly.

> **SUMMARY**
>
> Normal ECG, with prominent U waves.

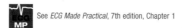 See *ECG Made Practical*, 7th edition, Chapter 1

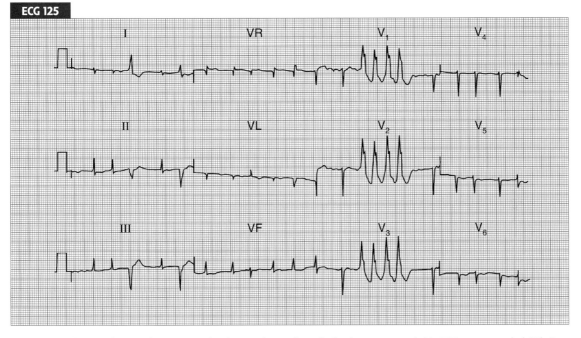

A 60-year-old man who was being treated in hospital complained of palpitations, and this ECG was recorded. What do you think the underlying disease was, and what were the palpitations due to?

ANSWER 125

The ECG shows:

- Atrial fibrillation
- Ventricular extrasystoles with two distinct morphologies (best seen in lead II)
- A four-beat run of ventricular tachycardia
- Right axis deviation
- Small QRS complexes
- No R wave development in the chest leads; lead V_6 shows a dominant S wave
- T wave inversion in leads V_5–V_6.

Clinical interpretation

This ECG suggests chronic lung disease – small complexes, right axis deviation and marked 'clockwise rotation', with lead V_6 still showing a right ventricular type of complex (i.e. a complex with a small R wave and a deeper S wave, as normally seen in lead V_1). The atrial fibrillation is probably secondary to the lung disease, although other possibilities must be considered. The patient's lung condition may be being treated with a beta-agonist, such as salbutamol, and this could be the cause of the extrasystoles and ventricular tachycardia.

What to do

Check the electrolyte levels. If the patient is taking a beta-agonist then reducing or stopping this, if possible, may help. If he does not have reversible airways disease a beta-blocker could be considered. Even with some lung diseases (such as COPD) a cardioselective beta-blocker can sometimes be tolerated. Alternatives for rate control would be a calcium channel-blocker or digoxin. Remember to assess for risks/hazards of anticoagulation as this is very likely to be indicated.

> **SUMMARY**
>
> Atrial fibrillation with ventricular extrasystoles and ventricular tachycardia; changes suggesting chronic lung disease.

 See *ECG Made Practical*, 7th edition, Chapters 4 and 7

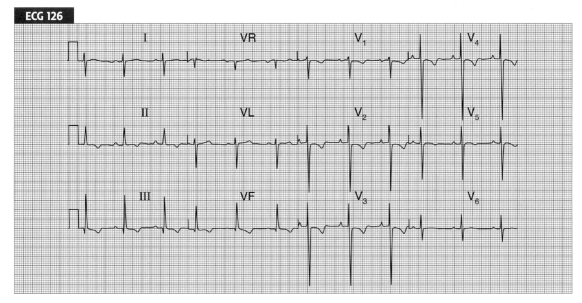

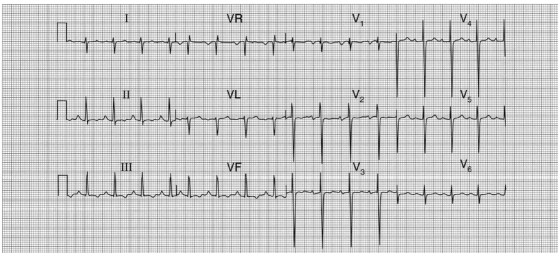

A 70-year-old man gave a history of several years of chest pain on exertion. These are his ECGs at rest (upper trace) and on exercise (lower trace). What do they show?

ANSWER 126

The upper ECG shows:
- Sinus rhythm, rate 68 bpm
- Right axis deviation
- Small Q waves in leads III, VF
- Persistent S wave in leads V_5–V_6
- Inverted T waves in leads II, III, VF, V_1–V_5.

The lower record was taken during stage 2 of the Bruce protocol. It shows:
- Sinus rhythm at 100 bpm
- T wave inversion persists in leads II, III, VF; but the T waves are now upright in the chest leads.

Clinical interpretation

Exercise testing is no longer a central element of guideline-based assessment of stable chest pain syndromes which now largely favour imaging-based investigations. However it is still performed in many centres. The widespread T wave inversion suggests a non-ST segment elevation myocardial infarction, although there is nothing in the history to suggest when this occurred. The S wave in lead V_6 suggests the possibility of chronic lung disease. The change in the T waves in the anterior leads, from inverted at rest to normal on exercise, is an example of 'pseudonormalization', which is an indication of ischaemia.

What to do

'Pseudonormalization' must be regarded in the same way as the usual ST segment response to ischaemia, which is depression. This patient's exercise test was positive (i.e. indicates ischaemia) at a relatively low level – he requires guideline-based treatment for ischaemic heart disease and anti-anginal therapy pending a coronary angiogram with a view to revascularization.

SUMMARY

Ischaemia with 'pseudonormalization' of the ECG on exercise.

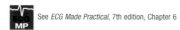

See *ECG Made Practical*, 7th edition, Chapter 6

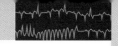

ECG 127

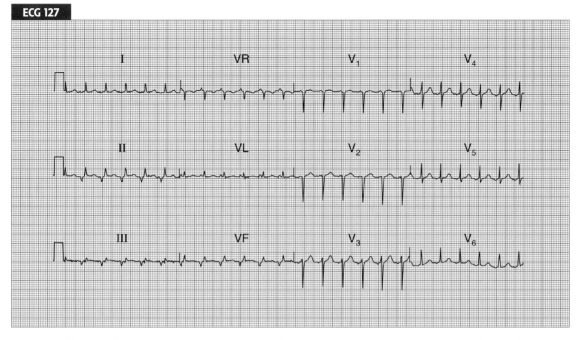

A 30-year-old man, who had complained of palpitations for many years without anything abnormal being found, came to the A&E department during an attack, and this ECG was recorded. Apart from signs of marked anxiety, there were no unusual findings except a heart rate of 140 bpm. What does the ECG show?

ANSWER 127

The ECG shows:
- Narrow complex tachycardia at 140 bpm
- Inverted P waves, most obvious in leads II, III, VF
- Short PR interval (about 100 ms)
- Normal axis
- Normal QRS complexes, ST segments and T waves.

Clinical interpretation

The story of attacks of palpitations could indicate episodes of sinus tachycardia due to anxiety, but the heart rate of 140 bpm suggests that a rhythm other than sinus rhythm is likely. This ECG clearly shows a supraventricular tachycardia of some sort, with one P wave per QRS complex. It could be sinus tachycardia, and the short PR interval could indicate pre-excitation, but the abnormal P waves in the inferior leads make this unlikely. This is either an atrial tachycardia or an AV-nodal re-entry tachycardia.

What to do

Increasing AV nodal conduction will help distinguish between an AVNRT (where this may terminate the attack) or atrial tachycardia (where this may reduce conduction to 2:1 or more). Carotid sinus massage or other vagal manoeuvres may be tried, but if not incremental doses of adenosine can be used. Treatment depends on the frequency of attacks. Further attacks may be prevented by a beta-blocker, but if frequent episodes persist an electrophysiological study should be considered.

SUMMARY

Atrial tachycardia.

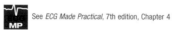 See *ECG Made Practical*, 7th edition, Chapter 4

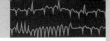

ECG 128

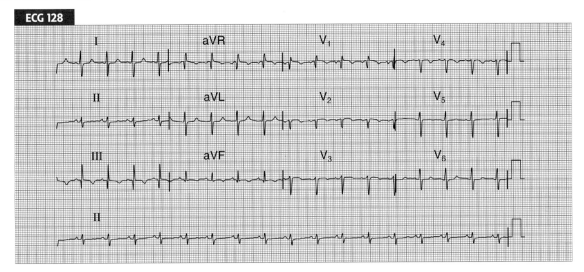

A 40-year-old man known to have angina develops chest pain 2 days after knee replacement surgery. Does his ECG help with the diagnosis?

ANSWER 128

The ECG shows:
- Sinus rhythm at 100 bpm
- Right axis deviation
- Q waves in lead 3
- "Clockwise rotation" with a persistent S wave in V_6
- Inverted T waves in leads 3, VF and V_1–V_4.

Clinical interpretation

Chest pain after knee surgery obviously raises the possibility of a pulmonary embolus, but this man had had previous angina so he might have had a myocardial infarction. Either would explain the sinus tachycardia. The Q wave in lead 3 with inverted T waves in leads 3 and VF could be due to ischaemia, but the right axis, clockwise rotation and inverted T waves in most of the chest leads would be more typical of a pulmonary embolus. This ECG shows the "S1 Q3 T3" combination often claimed to be typical of pulmonary embolism, but this pattern on its own is actually rare.

What to do

He needs a computed tomography (CT) pulmonary angiogram, and anti-coagulation after consultation with the surgeon.

> **SUMMARY**
>
> Sinus tachycardia, right axis, clockwise rotation and T wave inversion all suggestive of pulmonary embolism.

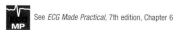 See *ECG Made Practical*, 7th edition, Chapter 6

ECG 129

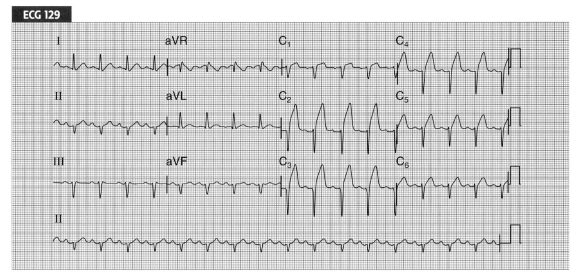

This ECG was recorded from a 50-year-old man admitted after 2 h of severe central chest pain. There are least four abnormalities.

ANSWER 129

The ECG shows:

- Sinus rhythm rate 110 bpm
- Left axis deviation
- Possible Q waves in leads V_3 and V_4
- Poor R wave development in the chest leads, with dominant S wave in lead V_6
- Raised ST segments $V_2–V_4$
- Peaked T waves, especially in leads $V_2–V_4$.

Clinical interpretation

This ECG shows an anterior ST-segment elevation myocardial infarction (STEMI). The peaked 'hyperacute' T waves suggest an acute process. The left axis might be new but could be old. A previous ECG, if available, would help here, but more importantly it would help to explain the loss of R waves the chest leads. The absent R waves could indicate an old anterior infarction, but the deep S waves in V_6 could be due to 'clockwise rotation', suggesting chronic lung disease.

What to do

Don't waste too much time trying to find a previous ECG! Treat as an acute STEMI and alert the cardiac catherterization team to prepare for a primary angioplasty case.

SUMMARY

Anterior STEMI with 'hyperacute' T waves, left axis and possible clockwise rotation due to chronic lung disease.

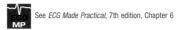 See *ECG Made Practical*, 7th edition, Chapter 6

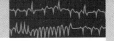

ECG 130

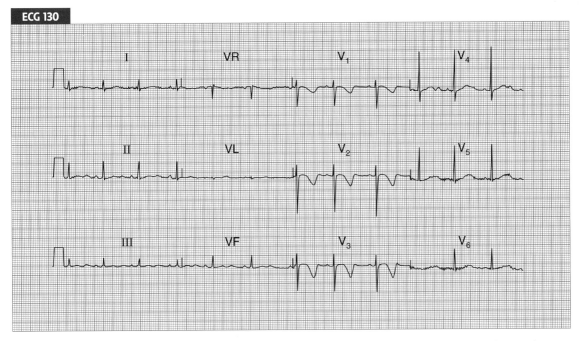

This ECG was recorded from a 15-year-old boy who collapsed while playing football, but was well by the time he was seen. What are the possible diagnoses?

ANSWER 130

The ECG shows:
- Sinus rhythm, rate 75 bpm
- Normal PR interval and QRS complex duration
- Normal axis
- Normal QRS complexes
- Inverted T waves in leads V_1–V_3
- Long QT interval (520 ms).

Clinical interpretation

A collapse during exercise raises the possibility of aortic stenosis, hypertrophic cardio-myopathy or an exercise-induced arrhythmia. This ECG does not show the pattern of left ventricular hypertrophy, so aortic stenosis is unlikely. Anterior T wave inversion is characteristic of hypertrophic cardiomyopathy, but this does not normally cause a prolonged QT interval. Exercise-induced arrhythmias are typical of the familial long QT syndrome, and this boy's sister had died suddenly.

What to do

Avoidance of drugs which prolong the QT interval or cause hypokalaemia or hypomag-nesaemia is essential (for example see https://www.crediblemeds.org/). Initial treatment is with a beta-blocker. Referral for family genetic testing is important. Specialist assessment is required for an ICD (implantable cardioverter defibrillator).

SUMMARY

The congenital long QT syndrome.

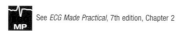 See *ECG Made Practical*, 7th edition, Chapter 2

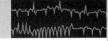

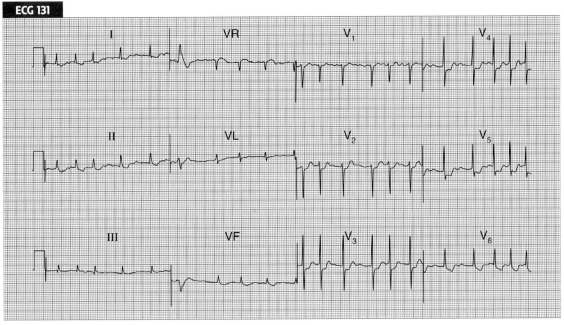

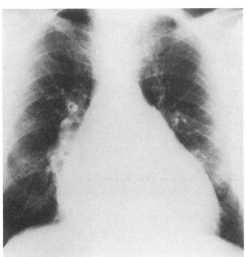

This ECG and chest X-ray are from a 60-year-old man being treated as an outpatient for severe congestive cardiac failure. What might be the diagnosis of the underlying heart condition, and what would you do?

ANSWER 131

The ECG shows:
- Atrial fibrillation
- Average ventricular rate 120 bpm
- Normal axis
- Normal QRS complexes
- Horizontal ST segment depression in leads V_3–V_4
- Downward-sloping ST segment depression in leads I, II, V_5–V_6.

The chest X-ray shows a generally enlarged heart, but especially an enlarged left ventricle and left atrium.

Clinical interpretation

The ventricular rate is not adequately controlled, though the downward-sloping ST segment depression suggests that he is taking digoxin. The horizontal ST segment depression suggests ischaemia.

What to do

Despite the ECG evidence of ischaemia, possible diagnoses include valvular heart disease, thyrotoxicosis, alcoholic heart disease and other forms of cardiomyopathy. The chest X-ray suggests severe mitral regurgitation. Echocardiography is necessary. In addition to treatments targeting a specific cause (e.g. consideration of valve surgery), the patient requires guideline-based treatment for heart failure, anticoagulation and improved rate control (probably by the cautious introduction or up-titration of a beta-blocker).

> **SUMMARY**
>
> Atrial fibrillation with an uncontrolled ventricular rate, probable ischaemia and digoxin effect.

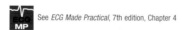 See *ECG Made Practical*, 7th edition, Chapter 4

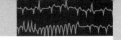

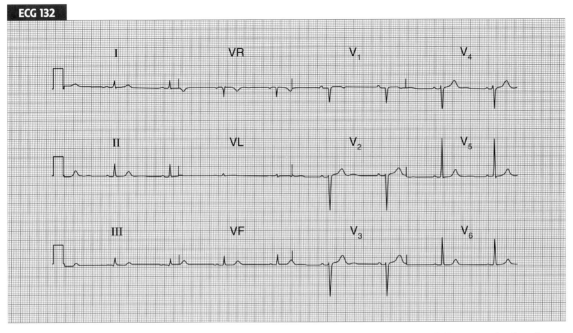

A 65-year-old man is seen in the outpatient department complaining of breathlessness and chest pain that has the characteristics of angina. He is untreated. Does his ECG help with his diagnosis and management?

ANSWER 132

The ECG shows:
- Sinus rhythm, rate 48 bpm
- Normal axis
- Small R waves in leads V_2–V_4 and a normal (tall) R wave in lead V_5.

Clinical interpretation

The small R waves in leads V_2–V_4 and the 'sudden' appearance of a normal R wave in lead V_5 is called 'poor R wave progression', and despite the absence of Q waves this probably indicates an old anterior infarction. An alternative explanation might be poor lead positioning.

What to do

The ECG should be repeated, to ensure proper positioning of the chest leads. An echocardiogram and a chest X-ray are needed, to see if left ventricular impairment is responsible for the breathlessness. Further investigation is also required for the chest pain for example by perfusion imaging or CT coronary angiography. Management will depend on the results of these investigations.

> **SUMMARY**
>
> Poor R wave progression, suggesting an old anterior myocardial infarction.

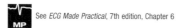 See *ECG Made Practical*, 7th edition, Chapter 6

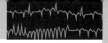

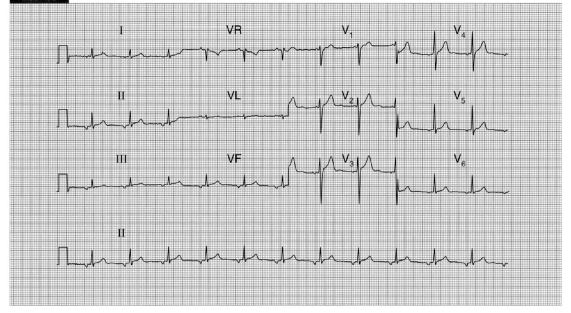

This ECG was recorded from a 30-year-old woman who complained of palpitations. Does it help in making a diagnosis?

ANSWER 133

The ECG shows:
- Ectopic atrial rhythm, with inverted P waves in leads II, III, VF, V_3–V_6; ventricular rate 69 bpm
- Normal axis
- Normal QRS complexes and T waves.

Clinical interpretation

This appears to be a stable rhythm originating in the atrial muscle rather than the sinoatrial (SA) node – hence the abnormal P wave and the slightly short PR interval (130 ms). This rhythm is not uncommon, and is usually of no clinical significance. It is unlikely to be the cause of her symptoms unless at times she has a paroxysmal atrial tachycardia.

What to do

Take a careful history and attempt to determine whether her symptoms sound like a paroxysmal tachycardia – ask about any sudden onset and ending of the palpitations; associated symptoms such as breathlessness; precipitating and terminating factors; and so on. If in doubt, some sort of ambulatory recording will be needed.

> **SUMMARY**
>
> Ectopic atrial rhythm.

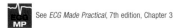 See *ECG Made Practical*, 7th edition, Chapter 3

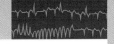

ECG 134

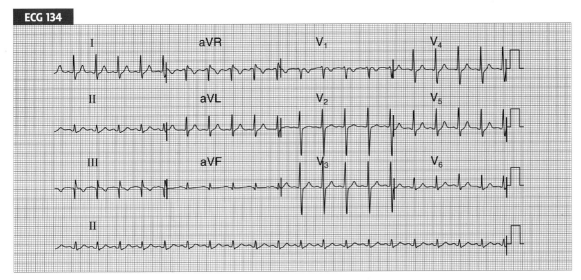

A 30-year-old woman, who had given birth 2 weeks previously, complained of breathlessness. Pulmonary embolism was obviously a possible diagnosis. Does the ECG help?

ANSWER 134

This ECG shows:
- Sinus rhythm rate 120 bpm
- Normal axis
- Q wave in lead III, but otherwise normal QRS complexes
- Inverted T wave in lead III but not elsewhere.

Clinical interpretation

The only definite abnormality in this recording is the sinus tachycardia, which could be due to many things including anxiety or anaemia. The Q wave in lead III with the inverted T wave could be a normal variant, and there are no indicators of right ventricular hypertrophy. However, the most common ECG finding in pulmonary embolism is sinus tachycardia without any other change, and the diagnosis must be made on clinical and imaging grounds, not on the ECG findings.

What to do

An echocardiogram may be helpful, but an urgent computed tomography (CT) pulmonary angiogram would be the investigation of choice following anticoagulation with a low molecular weight heparin.

SUMMARY

Sinus tachycardia; the Q and inverted T wave in lead III could be a normal variant.

 See *ECG Made Practical*, 7th edition, Chapters 6 and 7

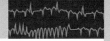

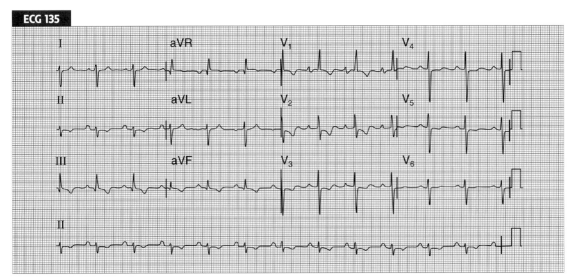

A 50-year-old woman has been becoming increasingly breathless over the past year. What are the possible diagnoses?

ANSWER 135

This ECG shows:
- Sinus rhythm, 80 bpm
- Right axis
- Dominant R wave of the QRS complex in lead V_1
- Dominant S wave in lead V_6
- Inverted T waves in leads V_1–V_3 with biphasic T waves in V_4–V_6.

Clinical interpretation

The peaked P waves suggest right atrial hypertrophy. The right axis, dominant R in V_1 and clockwise rotation, with inverted T waves in leads V_1–V_3 are the classic changes of right ventricular hypertrophy. This is not likely to be due to valve disease, and she almost certainly has either primary or chronic thromboembolic pulmonary hypertension.

What to do

An echocardiogram and computed tomography (CT) pulmonary angiogram will help with the diagnosis, but patients with primary pulmonary hypertension are best managed in a specialist unit.

> **SUMMARY**
>
> Right ventricular hypertrophy.

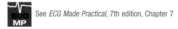 See *ECG Made Practical*, 7th edition, Chapter 7

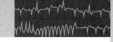

ECG 136

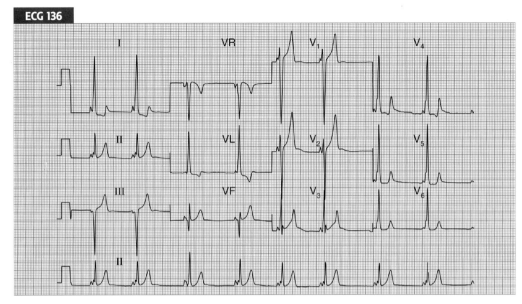

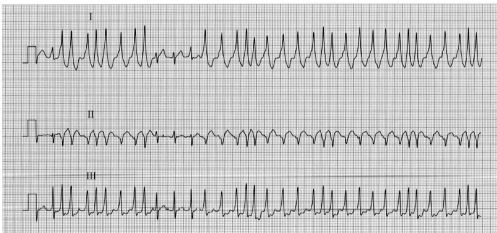

These ECGs were recorded from a 20-year-old man who had had attacks of a fast and irregular heartbeat for several years. The upper trace was recorded when he was asymptomatic; the lower trace (rhythm strips only) was recorded during one of his attacks. What is the diagnosis, and what would you do next?

275

ANSWER 136

The upper ECG shows:
- Sinus rhythm, rate 51 bpm
- Very short PR interval
- Normal axis
- Bizarre and widened QRS complexes with a slurred upstroke (delta wave), best seen in leads I and V_4–V_6.

The lower ECG shows:
- A very irregular tachycardia with a ventricular rate of up to 200 bpm
- No visible P waves
- A few normal complexes, but the majority are wide and have a slurred upstroke.

Clinical interpretation

This is the Wolff–Parkinson–White (WPW) syndrome: the accessory pathway is on the right side, and this is sometimes called 'type B'. The irregular tachycardia is due to atrial fibrillation.

What to do

Atrial fibrillation in the WPW syndrome can lead to sudden death due to ventricular fibrillation, so ablation of the abnormal pathway is needed urgently. Immediate treatment of the atrial fibrillation should be by cardioversion and flexainide can be used to protect against further pre-excited atrial fibrillation while definitive electrophysiological management is arranged. Digoxin, verapamil, beta blockers and diltiazem should be avoided because these block the atrioventricular node and encourage conduction through the accessory pathway.

SUMMARY

The WPW syndrome type B with paroxysmal pre-excited atrial fibrillation.

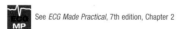 See *ECG Made Practical*, 7th edition, Chapter 2

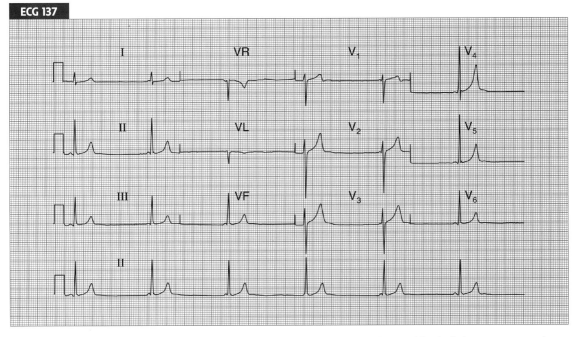

This ECG was recorded as part of the 'screening' examination of a young professional football player. Is it normal?

ANSWER 137

The ECG shows:

- Regular narrow complex rhythm at 35 bpm
- P waves sometimes, but not always, visible just before the QRS complexes
- PR interval, when measurable, is always short but varies
- Height of R wave in lead V_4 plus depth of S wave in lead V_2=49 mm
- Normal QRS complexes and ST segments
- Peaked T waves, especially in lead V_4.

Clinical interpretation

The short PR interval raises the possibility of pre-excitation, but the interval varies, and in the first complex of leads V_1–V_3 no P wave can be seen. The slow, narrow complex rhythm suggests atrioventricular nodal escape. Here there is a pronounced slowing of the sinoatrial node, presumably due to athletic training, and an accelerated idionodal rhythm has taken over. This pattern used to be called a 'wandering atrial pacemaker'. The tall R waves are perfectly normal in young fit people, and so are the peaked T waves.

What to do

This is a normal variant in athletes, and no action is required.

> **SUMMARY**
>
> Accelerated idionodal rhythm.

 See *ECG Made Practical*, 7th edition, Chapter 1

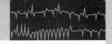

ECG 138

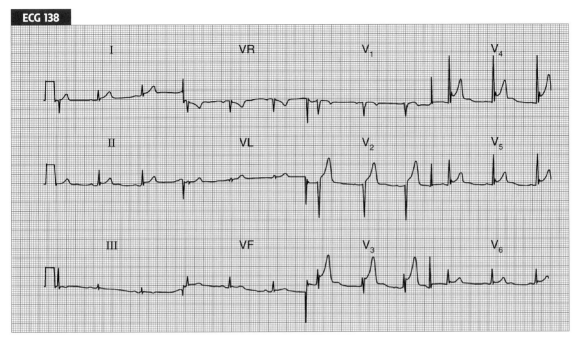

A 30-year-old man is seen in the A&E department with left-sided chest pain that appears to be pleuritic in nature. What does his ECG show?

ANSWER 138

The ECG shows:
- Sinus rhythm, rate 63 bpm
- Normal axis
- Normal QRS complexes
- Raised ST segments in leads II, V_3–V_6, in each case preceded by an S wave.

Clinical interpretation

When a raised ST segment follows an S wave as shown here, it is called 'high take-off' of the ST segment. This is a normal variant, which must be distinguished from the changes associated with an acute infarction or pericarditis.

What to do

If the patient has chest pain that appears to be pleuritic, then pulmonary rather than cardiac causes of pain should be considered – infection, pulmonary embolus and pneumothorax. The ECG is completely unhelpful here.

> **SUMMARY**
>
> Normal ECG showing 'high take-off' ST segment.

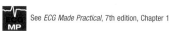 See *ECG Made Practical*, 7th edition, Chapter 1

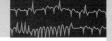

ECG 139

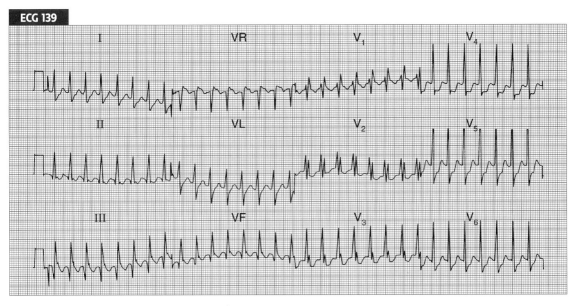

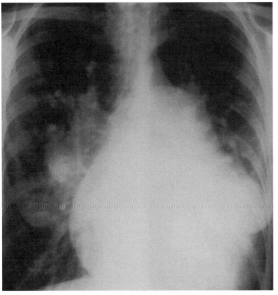

A 25-year-old man, known to have a heart problem for which he had refused surgery, was admitted to hospital as an emergency because of palpitations. His heart rate was 170 bpm, his blood pressure was 140/80 and there were no signs of heart failure. What is the cardiac rhythm, and what would you do?

ANSWER 139

The ECG shows:
- Rate 170 bpm
- No clear P waves but possibly some P waves visible in lead VR
- Normal axis
- QRS duration 120 ms
- Right bundle branch block (RBBB) pattern
- Horizontal ST segment depression, best seen in lead V_4.

The chest X-ray shows a very large heart with prominence of the right ventricle and pulmonary outflow, and large peripheral pulmonary arteries indicating a left-to-right shunt. These features are compatible with a large atrial septal defect.

Clinical interpretation

The QRS complex duration is 120 ms, the axis is normal and the QRS complexes show the classic RBBB pattern. It is likely that this is a supraventricular tachycardia with RBBB, and this diagnosis would be certain if we were sure of the existence of P waves in lead VR. This is either an atrial or an atrioventricular nodal re-entry (junctional) tachycardia (AVNRT). The ST segment depression suggests ischaemia.

What to do

If the patient has an atrial septal defect, he is likely to have RBBB, and this could be confirmed from pre-existing hospital records. The initial treatment is carotid sinus massage, and if this proves ineffective, intravenous adenosine. This will either terminate a re-entry tachycardia or increase AV-block to reveal an underlying atrial tachycardia.

SUMMARY

Supraventricular tachycardia (possibly atrial, possibly AVNRT) with RBBB; atrial septal defect.

 See *ECG Made Practical*, 7th edition, Chapter 4

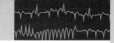

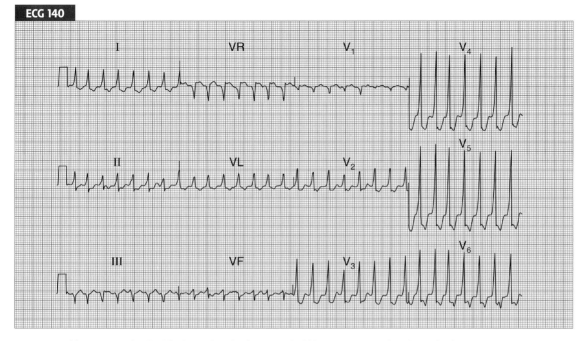

A 35-year-old woman, who had had attacks of what sounded like a paroxysmal tachycardia for many years, was seen in the A&E department, and this ECG was recorded. What is the diagnosis?

ANSWER 140

The ECG shows:

- Narrow complex tachycardia at about 170 bpm
- No P waves visible
- Normal axis
- QRS complex duration 112 ms
- Slurred upstroke to QRS complexes, best seen in leads V_3–V_6
- Depressed ST segments in leads V_3–V_6
- Inverted T waves in the lateral leads.

Clinical interpretation

This is a narrow complex tachycardia, so it is supraventricular. The slurred upstroke to the QRS complex suggests the Wolff–Parkinson–White (WPW) syndrome, so this is a re-entry tachycardia, with depolarization spreading down the accessory pathway. The absence of a dominant R wave in lead V_1 indicates that this is WPW syndrome type B. This diagnosis is consistent with the patient's history.

What to do

Carotid sinus pressure is always the first thing to try in patients with a supraventricular tachycardia. In most such patients, adenosine is the first drug to use provided you are absolutely certain the rhythm is not pre-excited atrial fibrillation (when adenosine could be dangerous). If in doubt DC cardioversion under sedation or anaesthesia is an alternative. An electrophysiological ablation procedure is the definitive management; in the interim drugs which block the atrioventricular node (such as beta blockers, calcium channel blockers and digoxin) should be avoided but flexainide can be used as prophylaxis against further arrhythmia.

SUMMARY

Supraventricular tachycardia and the WPW syndrome type B.

 See *ECG Made Practical*, 7th edition, Chapter 4

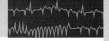

ECG 141

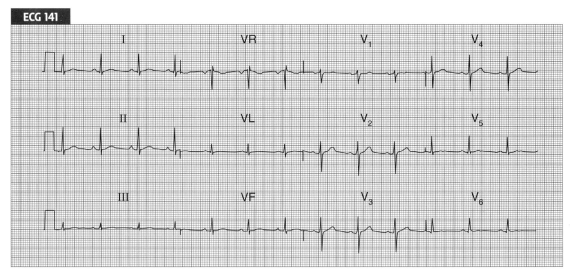

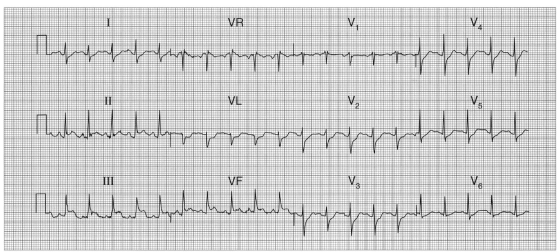

A 50-year-old man complains of pain in the front of his chest, which is predictably induced by walking uphill, especially in cold weather. The pain is sometimes caused by excitement. He has never had any pain without some precipitating cause. The upper ECG shows a recording made at rest, and the lower record comes from his exercise test, after 5 min of the Bruce protocol. What do the ECGs show?

ANSWER 141

Upper ECG

The upper ECG shows:

- Sinus rhythm with a rate of 75 bpm
- Normal axis
- Normal QRS complexes
- Normal ST segments
- Flat T wave in lead VL; flat and possibly biphasic T wave in lead V_6.

Clinical interpretation

The T wave changes are very nonspecific, and the trace could well be normal. However, since the patient's story is highly suggestive of angina, an exercise test is necessary.

Exercise test

The lower ECG shows:

- Sinus rhythm with a rate of about 110 bpm
- ST segment depression in leads V_2–V_4, with a maximum in lead V_3
- ST segment elevation in leads II, III, VF.

Clinical interpretation

The ST segment depression in leads V_2–V_4 is upward-sloping, so it does not allow a confident diagnosis of ischaemia. The ST segment elevation in leads II, III and VF is suggestive of an acute inferior myocardial infarction. In this case, the ST segment elevation cleared immediately on resting – elevation like this is an occasional manifestation of ischaemia rather than infarction.

What to do

This patient's exercise-ECG is very high risk and admission for urgent coronary angiography with a view to revascularization is indicated. In the interim he should be started on dual antiplatelet therapy and guideline-based management for ischaemic heart disease.

SUMMARY

Normal ECG at rest; ST segment elevation on exercise.

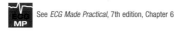 See *ECG Made Practical*, 7th edition, Chapter 6

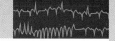

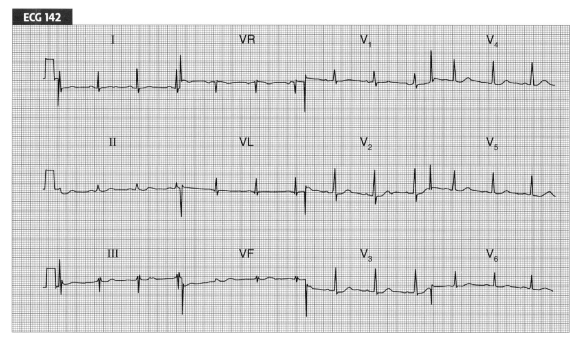

A 40-year-old man is seen in the outpatient department with a history that suggests a myocardial infarction 3 weeks previously. There are no abnormalities on examination, and this is his ECG. There are two possible explanations for the abnormality it shows, though only one of these would explain his history. What is the likely diagnosis?

ANSWER 142

The ECG shows:
- Sinus rhythm, rate 71 bpm
- Normal axis
- Dominant R waves in lead V_1
- ST segment depression in leads V_2–V_3
- Nonspecific T wave flattening in leads I, VL.

Clinical interpretation

The dominant R waves in lead V_1 might indicate right ventricular hypertrophy, but there are none of the other features that would be associated with this – right axis deviation, and T wave inversion in leads V_1, V_2 and possibly V_3. The changes are therefore probably due to a posterior myocardial infarction, which would fit the history of chest pain 3 weeks previously.

What to do

It is important not to miss a diagnosis of pulmonary embolism. The patient should be re-examined to ensure that there is no clinical evidence of right ventricular hypertrophy. A chest X-ray examination should be carried out, and an echocardiogram may be helpful. CT pulmonary angiography should be considered depending on the clinical suspicion.

SUMMARY

Probable posterior myocardial infarction.

 See *ECG Made Practical*, 7th edition, Chapter 6

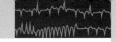

ECG 143

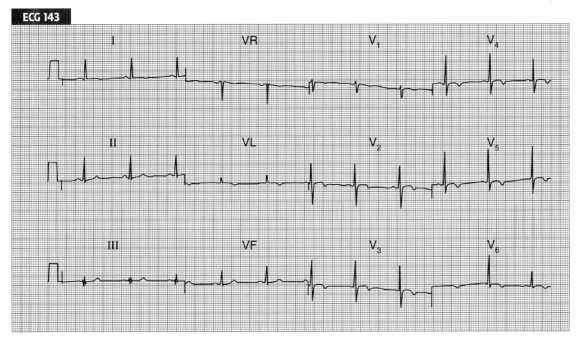

This ECG was recorded from a 55-year-old woman of African origin who had been complaining for several years of chest pain, and was admitted to hospital with persistent pain that was not characteristic of ischaemia. How would you have managed her?

ANSWER 143

The ECG shows:

- Sinus rhythm, rate 60 bpm
- Normal axis
- Normal QRS complexes; variation in the complexes in lead V_6 is probably due to an artefact
- T wave inversion in leads I, VL, V_2–V_6.

Clinical interpretation

With this history, an anterolateral non-ST segment elevation acute coronary syndrome has to be the first diagnosis, but T wave 'abnormalities' are common in people of African origin, and this ECG could be normal.

What to do

In this patient, the diagnosis of an acute infarction was excluded when the plasma high sensitivity troponin levels were found to be normal. An exercise test was performed, but was limited by breathlessness without further ECG change. A coronary angiogram was completely normal. The chest pain was therefore thought to be musculoskeletal in origin, and the T wave changes were presumably due to her ethnicity.

> **SUMMARY**
>
> Widespread T wave 'abnormalities', normal in a woman of African origin.

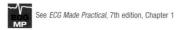 See *ECG Made Practical*, 7th edition, Chapter 1

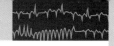

ECG 144

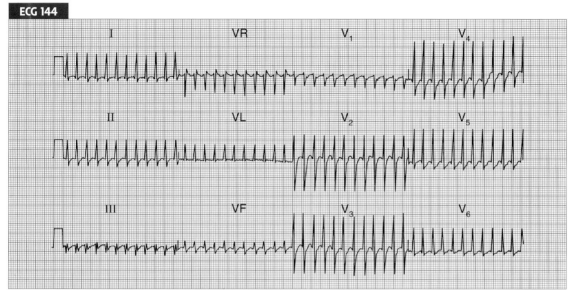

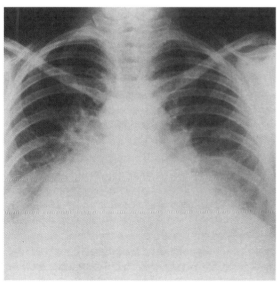

A 50-year-old man, who had complained of attacks of dizziness and palpitations for several years, collapsed at work and was brought to the A&E department. He was cold and clammy. His heart rate was rapid and his blood pressure was unrecordable. There were signs of left ventricular failure. These are his ECG and chest X-ray. What do they show and what would you do?

ANSWER 144

The ECG shows:
- Narrow complex tachycardia, rate just under 300 bpm
- No definite P waves
- Normal QRS complexes
- ST segment depression in leads V_4–V_6.

The chest X-ray shows pulmonary oedema.

Clinical interpretation

A regular narrow complex tachycardia at 300 bpm probably represents atrial flutter with 1:1 conduction (i.e. each atrial activation causes ventricular activation).

What to do

The cardiovascular collapse results from the rapid heart rate, with a loss of diastolic filling. As the patient is haemodynamically compromised by his tachycardia, he should be treated with immediate direct current (DC) cardioversion under sedation or anaesthesia.

SUMMARY

Probable atrial flutter with 1:1 conduction.

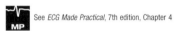 See *ECG Made Practical*, 7th edition, Chapter 4

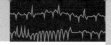

ECG 145

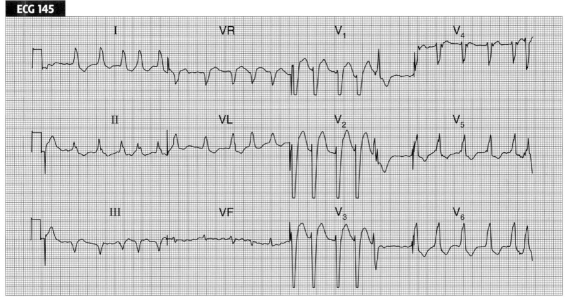

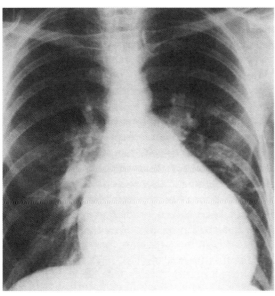

A 60-year-old man who complains of ankle swelling is found to have an irregular pulse, a blood pressure of 115/70, an enlarged heart, and signs of congestive cardiac failure. These are his ECG and chest X-ray. What do they show? He is untreated – how would you manage him?

ANSWER 145

The ECG shows:
- Atrial fibrillation, ventricular rate about 100 bpm, with one ventricular extrasystole
- Normal axis
- Broad QRS complexes, with 'M' pattern in the lateral leads indicating left bundle branch block (LBBB); bottom of S waves flattened in leads V_1–V_3 due to artefacts
- T waves inverted in lateral leads, as expected in LBBB.

The chest X-ray shows a very large heart, all chambers being affected, and there is upper-zone blood diversion, indicating early heart failure.

Clinical interpretation

Atrial fibrillation and LBBB in a patient with an enlarged heart.

What to do

This patient has had no chest pain, but has developed a very large heart with atrial fibrillation; the ECG shows LBBB, which prevents any further interpretation. Echocardiography will confirm a cardiomyopathy or may show a valvular cause. Other causes include ischaemia and alcohol or there may be no identifiable primary cause in 'idiopathic' dilated cardiomyopathy. The patient will require a careful workup to exclude primary causes and underlying coronary artery disease. Guideline-based treatment for heart failure should be initiated along with anticoagulation. Management may be complicated by his relatively low blood pressure. Given the broad QRS complex, device therapies e.g. cardiac resynchronization and defibrillator are also potentially indicated here.

> **SUMMARY**
>
> Atrial fibrillation and LBBB in a patient with dilated cardiomyopathy.

 See *ECG Made Practical*, 7th edition, Chapter 7

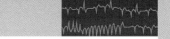

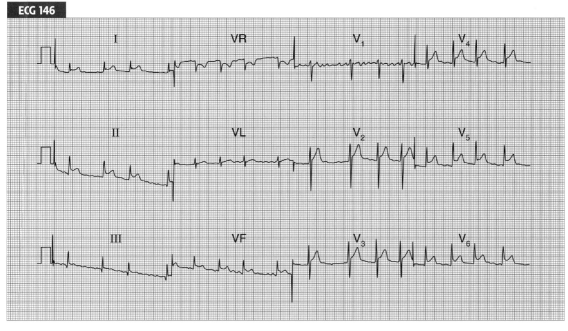

This ECG was recorded from a 30-year-old woman with severe rheumatoid arthritis, who was admitted to hospital with central chest pain. She was a non-smoker and had no risk factors for coronary artery disease. What do you think is going on?

ANSWER 146

The ECG shows:
- Atrial fibrillation, average rate about 100 bpm
- Normal axis
- Normal QRS complexes
- Raised ST segments in leads I, II, III, VF, V_2–V_6
- In leads V_3 and V_4 the raised ST segments seem to be due to 'high take-off'.

Clinical interpretation

In a young woman with chest pain but no risk factors for a myocardial infarction, an ST segment elevation infarction is obviously possible, but other causes of raised ST segments must be considered. The 'high take-off' ST segments in leads V_3–V_4 (raised ST segment following an S wave) are a normal variant. The other raised ST segments, which are widespread, could well be due to pericarditis.

What to do

The patient should be examined lying flat, because this gives the best chance of hearing a pericardial friction rub – and this is what was found here. The pericarditis could, of course, be due to an infarction, but repeated ECGs showed no development of an infarction pattern, and the raised ST segments persisted for several days. An echocardiogram showed a pericardial effusion. The pericarditis, and presumably the associated atrial fibrillation, were due to the rheumatoid arthritis. Initial management should be with non-steroidal anti-inflammatory drugs and colchicine. Early involvement of a rheumatologist would be recommended.

SUMMARY

Atrial fibrillation; ST segment elevation, partly 'high take-off' but mainly due to pericarditis.

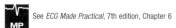 See *ECG Made Practical*, 7th edition, Chapter 6

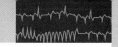

ECG 147

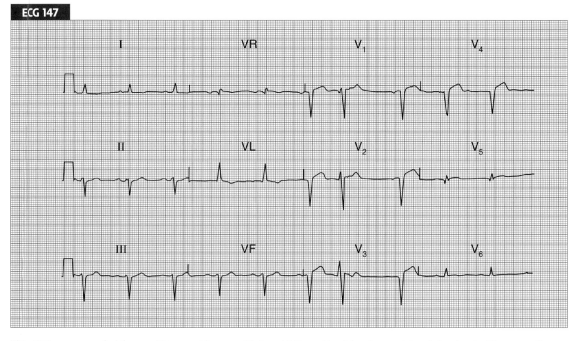

This ECG was recorded from a 75-year-old man with heart failure. He did not complain of chest pain. There are three main abnormalities. How should he be treated?

ANSWER 147

The ECG shows:
- Sinus rhythm, rate 60 bpm, with one ventricular extrasystole
- Left axis deviation
- Q waves in leads V_1–V_5 in the sinus beats
- Raised ST segments in the anterior leads
- Inverted T wave in lead VL; flattened T waves in leads I, V_6.

Clinical interpretation

A 'silent' anterior infarction of uncertain age has caused left anterior hemiblock, which explains the left axis deviation. The lateral T wave changes are presumably due to ischaemia.

What to do

Ventricular extrasystoles should not be treated, and left anterior hemiblock is not an indication for pacing. The clinical presentation and the presence of anterior Q waves suggest the anterior infarction is not new, so percutaneous coronary intervention (PCI) or thrombolysis should not be given. He needs echocardiography and guideline-based heart failure management.

SUMMARY

Left anterior hemiblock and anterior infarction of uncertain age; one ventricular extrasystole.

 See *ECG Made Practical*, 7th edition, Chapter 6

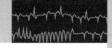

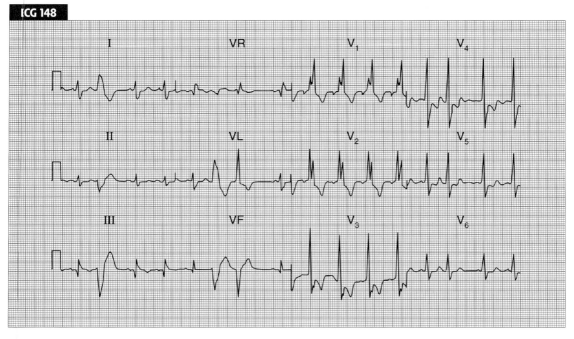

ICG 148

This ECG was recorded from a 65-year-old man who complained of breathlessness and who showed the physical signs of moderate heart failure. What does the ECG show? Does it have implications for treatment?

ANSWER 148

The ECG shows:
- Sinus rhythm, rate 97 bpm
- Multifocal ventricular extrasystoles and one supraventricular extrasystole
- Q waves in the sinus beats in leads III, VF
- Right bundle branch block (RBBB).

Clinical interpretation

The presence of Q waves in the inferior leads suggests an old infarction. Ischaemic disease is therefore probably the cause of the extrasystoles and the RBBB.

What to do

Control of the heart failure may well cause the extrasystoles to disappear; the extrasystoles should not be treated with antiarrhythmic drugs. He requires echocardiography and guideline-based heart failure management.

SUMMARY

Multifocal ventricular extrasystoles, RBBB and probable old inferior myocardial infarction.

 See *ECG Made Practical*, 7th edition, Chapter 6

ECG 149

ICG 149

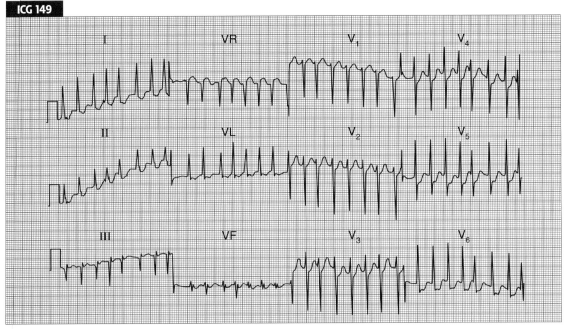

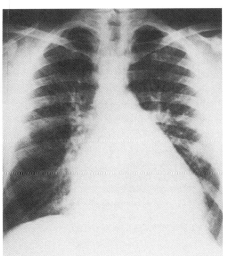

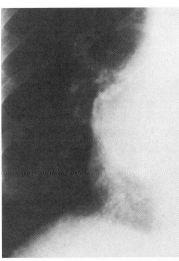

A 50-year-old woman came to the A&E department because of the sudden onset of palpitations and severe breathlessness. What abnormalities do the ECG and chest X-rays show, and what condition might be responsible? The X-ray on the right shows an enlargement of a penetrated view of the right heart border.

ANSWER 149

The ECG shows:
- Atrial fibrillation
- Normal axis
- Irregular QRS complexes with a ventricular rate of up to 200 bpm
- Otherwise normal QRS complexes, apart from an RSR[1] pattern in lead VF
- ST segments depressed in leads V_4–V_6, suggesting ischaemia
- Normal T waves.

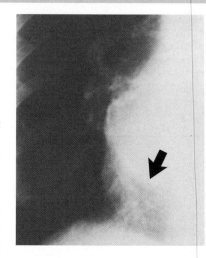

The chest X-ray shows an enlarged heart with a straight left heart border, which is due to left atrial (LA) enlargement. LA enlargement also causes a double shadow near the right heart border (arrowed).

Clinical interpretation

Atrial fibrillation with an uncontrolled ventricular rate. The ischaemic changes in leads V_4 and V_5 are probably related to the heart rate.

What to do

Ischaemia may have been the cause of the atrial fibrillation, or the rapid ventricular rate itself may be responsible for the ischaemic changes. Ischaemia is not a likely primary diagnosis in a 50-year-old woman, and the things to think about are valvular heart disease (particularly with mitral valve disease), thyrotoxicosis, alcoholism and other forms of cardiomyopathy. Immediate treatment of the heart failure with diuretics may be necessary, but the ventricular rate can be controlled initially by digoxin, given intravenously if necessary. Direct current (DC) cardioversion may be necessary if the patient is in severe heart failure. Remember that a patient with atrial fibrillation probably needs anticoagulants on a long-term basis. Echocardiography confirmed that this patient had mitral stenosis.

SUMMARY

Atrial fibrillation with a rapid ventricular rate and ischaemic changes, in a patient with mitral stenosis.

 See *ECG Made Practical*, 7th edition, Chapter 4

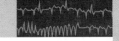

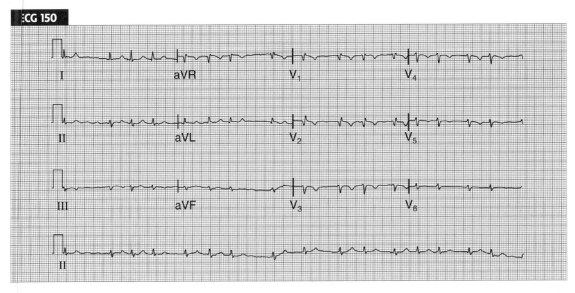

This ECG was recorded from an 80-year-old woman who had been in hospital for 3 weeks with a chest infection and heart failure. What does her ECG show?

ANSWER 150

The ECG shows:
- Atrial fibrillation, ventricular rate about 100 bpm
- Normal axis
- Low voltage QRS complexes
- Partial right bundle branch block; persistent S wave in V_6
- Inverted T waves V_1–V_5.

Clinical interpretation

This ECG has deliberately been chosen as the last one in the book because it is difficult to interpret and there is plenty of room for discussion. The record is properly calibrated so there should be an explanation for the small complexes: a pericardial effusion or chronic lung disease would be possibilities. The atrial fibrillation is presumably related to her heart failure, but without a previous ECG it is impossible to tell whether it is of recent onset. The partial right bundle branch block is not helpful for a diagnosis, but the persistent S wave in V_6 would fit with chronic lung disease. The most difficult features of this ECG are the inverted T waves in V_1–V_5. These could suggest an anterior non-ST segment elevation myocardial infarction (NSTEMI), but the most marked changes are in V_1–V_2 and therefore suggest a pulmonary embolus: this would be our preferred explanation.

What to do

Stop and think. Start again, taking a detailed medical history, examine the patient. Echocardiography, a chest X-ray and potentially CT pulmonary angiography may help tease out the differential diagnosis.

SUMMARY

Multiple abnormalities of uncertain cause.

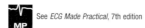 See *ECG Made Practical*, 7th edition

Index

Page numbers followed by "*f*" indicate figures.

305